What other physicians and authors say about
RENEWAL
Finding your path to self-healing in cancer

"The message we all need to receive is that cancer is not the end of our life but the beginning of a new life. Read *Renewal-Finding your path to self-healing in cancer* and learn how to live the authentic life intended for you."

-Bernie Siegel, MD,
author of *Love, Medicine & Miracles, 365 Prescriptions for The Soul*, etc.

"No one stands alone. No one should fall alone. Claude's wonderful testament to the near infinite renewal capacity inherent in Nature finds tender display in these stories of courage and caring. Read and rejoice."

-Walter M. Bortz II, MD,
author of *Dare to Be 100, We Live Too Short and Die Too Long*, etc.

"The stories told here provide the reader with a multifaceted view of living with (and dying from) cancer. Patients, friends and family, and health care professionals will find stories and concepts with which they can identify. Furthermore, patients may gain courage and strength from reading the experiences of others. This work introduces the reader to mechanisms to cope with a cancer diagnosis. It is truly empowering. I personally feel privileged to get to know some of the patients cared for by Dr. DeShazo and his team. I will recommend this book to my patients and to other doctors."

-David A. Kooby, MD, Winship Cancer Institute-Emory University,
Dept. of Surgery/Division of Surgical Oncology

Simon,

Renewal

Finding your path to self-healing in cancer

You are a comrade in many ways.
I hope you enjoy the book.

Semper Fi,

Claude V. DeShazo M.D.

Jan 10, 2010

Claude V. DeShazo, M.D.

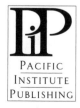

PACIFIC
INSTITUTE
PUBLISHING

Pacific Institute Publishing
1709 Harbor Avenue SW, Seattle, Washington 98126-2049
www.thepacificinstitute.com

ISBN 978-1-930622-16-6

3   5   7   9   10   8   6   4   2

Printed in Canada

TABLE OF CONTENTS

Renewal

---------- FOREWORD BY
BERNIE SIEGEL, M.D. ----------

I began support groups for people with cancer, and other serious illnesses, over thirty years ago. I offered them as an opportunity to help my patients live a longer better life when one said to me that she needed to know how to live between office visits.

Claude reminds me of my feelings and the lack of any opportunity to share them at medical meetings. The support groups I have been running for over thirty years are my therapy too. When I accept my mortality I empower myself. I have learned to live the message and enjoy my life's time. If I did not live what I preach I would find it very hard to continue to run support groups.

It took me many years to see that when people accepted their mortality and chose a new path for their lives, one their heart desired, it affected their survival and even lead to many examples of self-induced healing. We must remember our body loves us but if we do not give it love messages related to how we feel about our lives it responds in ways which will shorten the life we do not want to live. Monday morning with its increased frequency of heart attacks, strokes, suicides and illnesses speaks that message.

This is not about guilt, blame and shame but about understanding that one's feelings are communicated to your body. Our mind and bodies are one interactive unit. One cannot separate self from life experience. Studies show that loneliness affects the gene which controls immune function thus leading to more cases of cancer, infections and auto-immune diseases. Feeling loved or not by one's parents also predicts the likelihood of living a long healthy life. When confronted with a serious illness all these issues need to be looked at. We need to create the authentic life we choose for ourselves.

How can we turn a curse into a blessing? The ultimate message, portrayed by religions, myths and fairy tales is to be born again. When we are born again to a new life we choose and which eliminates what is killing us some wonderful things happen. We are all mortal and I am not talking about denying death or seeing it and not being cured of our disease as a failure. I am talking about taking on the challenge of life, making changes so that you can truly enjoy the time you have left and seeing that there are many labor pains involved in it but they all become worthwhile when one gives birth to a beloved child or your beloved self.

I bring this all up because I do not think that it is a coincidence, to quote DeShazo's words, "Along the way the group selected its own name, Renewal: A way towards healing." There are many ways to say one is born again and renewal is one of them. Just as a graduation is called a commencement and not a termination and the Bible ends in a revelation and not a conclusion so one can see life's problems as a choice for healthy growth and renewal.

Despite the fact that those who attend are facing life threatening illnesses I find there is more life, joy, love and tears when we meet and that one always goes home feeling uplifted because of the people who attend. They are very special and become guides and coaches for each other. For the most part doctors are tourists who do not understand that one doesn't live a diagnosis. One lives an experience and when we treat the experience and the patient's life we also help them to heal their lives and their disease as a by-product. They are an empowered group and not submissive sufferers.

There are personality characteristics to people who exceed expectations and that is what the Renewal group and ECaP portray. So read on and learn from their stories. When you provide the inspiration the information can lead to some wonderful results. You just have to show up for practice and that is what the Renewal groups keep doing. They act as if they are the person they want to become then rehearse and practice until they achieve their desires with the help of the group members who coach them through criticism, feedback and example.

The message we all need to receive is that cancer is not the end of our life but the beginning of a new life. Read Renewal and learn how to live the authentic life intended for you.

Peace,
Bernie

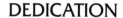

DEDICATION

This book is dedicated to the current and former members of the Renewal cancer support group in Kirkland, Washington. Their courage and dedication to helping themselves and one another inspire everyone around them. They certainly inspire me. These members are excited to share their experiences with a larger audience.

The book also is dedicated to one other person, my wife Maureen. For nearly forty years she has been an unflagging supporter, adviser, and inspiration in everything I do. For years she was an important but peripheral part of making Renewal activities successful. Then, in 2004, she earned the right to become a full-fledged member. Her personal experience with cancer brought her to a new level of understanding, contributed further to the group, and brought the two of us closer in our relationship.

ACKNOWLEDGMENTS

The value of this book is primarily vested in the stories Renewal members have written about themselves or related to me. Without these accounts this would be just another book about illness and treatment. Every member I called upon made a valuable contribution to what is here. This is especially true of Mr. John Barnett who made many valuable suggestions as well as writing a chapter about his experiences. Mrs. Rose Butler contributed much time locating members who moved away and gathering details. My agent, Barbara Neighbors Deal, was always available to share her vast knowledge of a complex publishing world with me.

At an early stage a retired editor, Mr. Wesley Curry, helped me focus on the essential theme of the manuscript and provided refinements. Over time Wes revealed his special insight came from being a cancer survivor himself.

My assistant Ms. Gilda Ignacio gave ongoing technical support and advice. She reduced the frustrations of composition to almost nothing.

Once again I have been fortunate enough to be able to call upon the talent of my daughter, Yvonne DeShazo, in doing art work. My son, Stephen DeShazo, provided valuable advice and research as work proceeded. The family contribution was rounded out by my wife, Maureen McGrade DeShazo, taking a turn at proofreading and clarifying some of the things I was attempting to say.

Mrs. Diane Tice and the staff of The Pacific Institute were extremely helpful in the final stages of bringing this book into being. This includes Mr. Jack Fitterer, Ms. Christy Watson, and Ms. Courtney Cook Hopp who did the final layout.

Claude V. DeShazo, M.D.
Carlsbad, California
March, 2009

CHAPTER 1
THE MEETINGS

"Put down the weight of your aloneness...
Everything is waiting for you."
— David Whyte, *Everything is Waiting for You*

It is late afternoon and outside the one-story building shadows lengthen on a garden of plants and flowers. There is a small stream, a pool, and a splashing fountain. Inside the building a wide bank of windows separates a well-lit conference room from this outside scene. A group of 30 men and women sit on chairs drawn into a circle.

A woman seated in the circle has just started to speak. She does not notice a tissue she twists with her hands has become moist and is beginning to fray. "I've been coming here now for several weeks." She pauses and readjusts to face two women seated to her left, "This is my fourth time." Each of the women she addresses has spoken about themselves just a few moments ago so the appearance is one of a conversation. The woman speaking continues as if addressing only these two, "I've been listening to the troubles all of you are having, but really didn't think I had anything to say." These past weeks, when invited to speak, the woman just shook her head and kept silent.

The speaker looks haggard and nervous but now seems determined to explain herself. She recounts the discovery of her cancer last year. Treatment is ongoing. Around the circle several others begin to nod their heads knowingly in agreement with what she says. The woman stops twisting the tissue in her hands. She surveys the rest of the group circle, seeming to make a last determination before revealing something. "So that's what's been going on with me. I've lived alone since my husband left. There isn't anyone else except my son." The pause is long, "And he's in prison." She waits, glancing down at her knees then back up, scanning the faces around her again. There is no movement, no perceptible change, so she continues, "He's been in there for two years. I go to see him whenever I get a chance." She speaks a little faster now as if wanting to finish, "It was for robbery and somebody got hurt… he's supposed to be in there for another five years."

Still nobody speaks. The woman's face suddenly crinkles. Tears make her eyes sparkle, "I don't know what to do about him." Tears are running down her cheeks, "I'm so ashamed!"

After a pause another woman across the room speaks softly but firmly, "It isn't your fault."

The woman who has been telling her story looks up, tracing the source of this unexpected comment. She dabs at her eyes and stops crying.

"He'll do his time and have to start over when he gets out," says a man in the group. He gives a nod as he speaks, suggesting some personal experience. "You have to let him find his way." He looks directly at the woman, "What you need to do now is take care of yourself."

Around the circle most of the heads begin to nod in agreement with this last comment. Members of the group sense that after these weeks of silence the woman speaking has released her great secret. This is the something that held back her participation. Several others offer anecdotes from their experience these comments have brought to mind. The group's facilitator makes a comment identifying several others in the room known to have this woman's same type of cancer. An exchange about experiences with treatment evolves and the conversation shifts to a more clinical theme.

That discussion ends and attention turns to the man seated next in the circle. He begins to speak about his own situation. The woman who has just finished revealing her secret is silent again but is visibly relieved. Her dark imaginings of being rejected because of her son's crime are ameliorated. She looks up, not down, and follows the sequence of reports given by others. She ventures several comments as the conversation moves around the circle, attention focusing first on one person then the next.

This interaction exemplifies much of what the group Renewal is about. The conversation above could have been any time during the years we've met or now. The impact of serious illness confronts people every day.

Let's jump right in. Here is Renewal from the members' perspective. As an exercise one Monday we spent the meeting getting clarity about why people were there. I as moderator asked for input. Here are quotes from the conversation that day with people saying what they wanted:

- I want to know, is conventional treatment enough?
- I've become confused. I've come here to sort these things out.
- I want more structure. I want psychological help because I don't think conventional treatment is enough.
- I want to know.....
- What I've learned is....
- I'm angry!
- I don't have cancer but it's in my family. It might happen to me.
- I want to learn how to live with cancer.
- I'm looking for a better source of information.
- My physician is not a source of hope. I want some group hope, group faith. I want to avoid negative behavior.
- I like to be comforted, have support and acceptance, and to let go!
- I'm concerned about whether I will "make it" or just die.
- I'm told my situation is hopeless; therefore I must look for alternatives.
- Where do I look for alternatives?
- What I thought I knew is all changing.
- Is it easier to be the person who is ill or the one living with someone who is ill?
- My husband has immune deficiency [with his cancer]. He puts up a good fight just to protect his job.
- How do we keep a [family] life going?
- How can I live with chemotherapy?
- I want to learn about the mind-body connection.
- Until I came here I had only met one person who survived cancer.
- [With indignation] What do you expect from us, miracles?
- [From a member who read a lot] What will bring about healing and personal transformation? I want to catch the "bloom of the present moment" [Thoreau].

How is that for defining the problems? And all in one afternoon! We might plausibly take this list as an outline for creating the rest of the book. In a way I have, but most answers come out in the personal stories of Renewal members, not from me. These are the issues; these were the kind of things on people's minds. That day was years ago but these are still pertinent comments and questions. They are what this book is about.

We need to preface our story by reminding ourselves of the rarity of support groups for cancer patients thirty years ago. Information about illnesses such as cancer was surprisingly hard to obtain except for what a doctor might tell you. And that might be, "This is your diagnosis; here is your treatment." That guidance might be pretty much all you'd get.

A person usually decides either to follow directions and receive the accolade of being a "good" patient, or be relegated to some category of "other." What we are going to explore in this book, mostly by example, is how consequences of this choice play out.

—⁂—

First, let's go back and look a bit more at how this all got started. I was well established in my practice of general surgery by the late 1970s. This practice, and that of my partners, included a high proportion of patients with cancers. In 1980 I served as Chief of the Medical Staff at my local hospital, just after finishing a stint as Chief of Surgery. Good as life was, I had two principle sources of dissatisfaction in what I was doing.

One was just plain working too hard. I was on the go day and night, keeping myself on the front line all the time. All this hurry and work caused the second problem. There was never enough time to spend with patients with serious medical problems at the very moment they appeared open to more advice.

One of the great things about a career as a surgeon is that when you demonstrably put your heart into it, a bond forms with many patients. They know when you are trying hard. They respect you; they will honor what you say. People like this really want to know what you think about their chances. "What do you think my prognosis is?" they ask, "What should I do?" If your personal experience causes you to doubt what I am saying, at least be open to the idea that serious illness creates teachable moments, opportunities for commitment and change.

This brings up the old adage about breakfast: the chicken laying the eggs is involved, but the pig supplying the bacon is committed. In cancer treatment the more dire a surgical situation, the greater the risk of losing body parts, normal function, or self image, the more likely a person is to become committed, not just involved. Still, commitment doesn't matter if it doesn't last. It is possible nothing will be learned and nothing gained. The opportunity recedes and becomes lost.

Commitment as I experienced it often appeared during a first post-op visit. Inquiry began with, "What should I do now?" Or more specifically, "What can I do to help myself?" In that instant we had entered a teachable moment. It was a chance for change and growth and what we came to call renewal. We had an opportunity to do something more and make a difference. I had a chance to seize that moment. Over time I learned to use that opening and work with it for a positive result.

Prior to Renewal I offered other options. One was a collection of pertinent books I could lend to patients who asked for more information. There really was a dearth of information available to the layman. What was there was too technical for most people. Even a library of medical journal reprints such as compiled by the Planetree Project at one San Francisco hospital was sparse. I tried to duplicate that approach locally but it wasn't feasible. Remember, this was before widespread use of the internet. So during that time I kept books and articles on exercise, stress reduction, yoga, diet and how it affected illness—anything I could find—and let patients borrow them.

Another accommodation frequently disrupted my clinic schedule. When I sensed a patient had come to a teachable moment, I tried to sit down, open a new dialogue, and stay in the moment. I asked what that person wanted, then listened to whatever and however the response came out. I asked more questions, clarifying intent, until I felt I understood a person's issues. Contrary to what you might expect from a surgeon, if a patient indicated in some way they felt they just were not ready to have an operation (in a pre-op visit), I'd support that. I'd say, "Fine, let's schedule another appointment in a week or two and go over this again."

Often, after concluding a conversation this way, a patient left the office only to call back a short time later. They'd leave a message to go ahead and schedule surgery. Or they'd want me called to the phone to tell me the same thing. Some of it was the reticence anyone has about surgery. In my opinion, another part of what was going on was a test to see how I would handle a rebuff of my professional advice. Some patients just needed a little breathing room to think. Still others needed to test how much control he or she could maintain in a fluid, high stakes situation. Dealing with cancer patients is not about having a script or planning what to say. This is about serendipity and listening. What really is being said? It is about being open to the moment and living every second of it.

When opportunities such as this arose I disregarded my tightly planned schedule. If I were living the kind of life I wanted to live on such days, I focused on that one patient no matter how long it took. My nurses and receptionists, overhearing that I was at it again, would start working the phones. They called appointments for later in the day to create space. They explained I was running behind schedule; please delay your arrival. Bless them. I didn't appreciate anything about time management. I know I was not assertive about staying in control of my time. I enjoyed the tension of give and take. Sometimes the conversation was raw, trying to break through and make connection with what that one patient needed at that very moment. For years I stopped wearing a wristwatch. I began hospital rounds early each day, then either went to the operating room or my clinic. I just kept working until everything was done.

Late in 1981 something fortunate happened. The University of Washington sponsored a weekend symposium. The symposium had a catchy title which I have long since forgotten. What I do remember about the Saturday session was two presentations, one by Dr. Larry Dossey and the other by Dr. Bernie Siegel. Larry still practiced as an internist in Dallas and Bernie as a general surgeon in New Haven, Connecticut. These two were heralds of a new attitude toward delivery of medical care, especially in cases with no easy fixes and the outcome in doubt. Both get more coverage later, but I want to emphasize here what Bernie did for me. He was able to express thoughts I had about not being able to share with cancer patients everything I knew. These were the patients who were searching. They wanted more information and more guidance. They especially wanted someone to be a co-traveler with them in the scariest journey they had ever undertaken.

Bernie gave a novel interpretation of how most people were conditioned to just follow along with medical advice, even if they had misgivings. A smaller number were open to helping themselves if it wasn't too hard or inconvenient. It was only the exceptional patients, maybe 10 to 15 per cent, who really wanted to get involved in their recovery. These people would try almost anything. These are the ones Bernie called his Exceptional Cancer Patients.

After the symposium I invited Bernie and his wife Bobbi to go out to dinner with my wife Maureen and me. We spent several hours talking about the very things that would lead Bernie to found the exceptional cancer patients (ECaP) groups soon thereafter. Bernie was, and still is, a dynamic speaker who had inspired thousands. He is the author of several successful books starting with *Love, Medicine, and Miracles*. When that book came out in 1986 it caused me to conclude that Bernie had written the definitive work and said all that needed to be said. This was the rationalization I used to shelve my own ideas of writing on the subject. Only now, 25 years later, am I finally putting down what I have to say and writing the Renewal story.

Love, Medicine, and Miracles was not published at that time in 1980, but the importance of what Bernie shared did come across to me. The takeaway message for me was, "Here is another general surgeon working every day just like me." He's in private practice, not sequestered in an ivory tower dreaming up ideas to perpetuate some research project. He was doing something outside the norm to support his patients. The conclusion I reached was, "Well, I have no idea how this will turn out, but if Bernie can do it, I can too."

Back at the office I went over my private list of surgical cases from the past year. I picked out the names of about three dozen people I could remember who had either asked me for some extra help or seemed interested in learning about their illness. In our conversations these were the people willing to be proactive about their health if only they knew what to do.

This book is about those people. Their troubles center on health matters coming suddenly to the fore as the most important issue in their lives. These people with many others comprise the membership of what became our cancer support group. What happens to our members became recognized as a renewal of who we are and what life means. Along the way the group self-selected its name, *Renewal: A way toward healing.*

The group actually had origin shortly before the Renewal meetings began in early 1982. I had been affected by the courageous fight of one of my patients against his colon cancer, his gradual acceptance of it, and his eventual death. This personal experience brought a number of issues to the surface and made me aware of new things. It became a tipping point.

I came to realize, more slowly than I like to admit, surgery ultimately is not everything. It dawned on me that my craft and conventional medical treatments in general sometimes are not everything hoped for by patients either.

—m—

DIXON (DICK). As I will do in the pages ahead, I call attention to some of the real people who made Renewal. The truth is, they made me. Just by being who they were and facing difficult situations with ingenuity, persistence, or grace (or all three and more) they are the real story of this book. Dixon, or Dick as most people called him, is the first of these even though he did not live long enough to come to a single Renewal meeting. Without his personal courage, I don't think I would have taken down my last barrier. Part of me was saying, "Be reasonable. Be practical. Don't try to pile more challenges onto the work you already are doing." I was intelligent enough back then, but not as wise as I became later. Now I can reflect on how Dick's life affected me in the years he was my patient. He personifies what overcame my reticence and got me going; that's why his story comes first.

Dick worked in construction, had his own business in partnership with a friend. He was about forty-five when I met him. He was noticeably quiet and soft spoken, not very likely to speak at all unless you asked him a direct question. He was not very tall but unusually strong. He was tough like a man becomes when he spends his whole life doing carpentry and plumbing and driving equipment. Unfortunately this toughness and unwillingness to complain is what got Dick into deep trouble. Dick's family physician had sent him over. Dick had gone in because, "Something might be wrong." His bowels had become irregular for a couple of years, then his bowel movements got smaller in diameter. The pain he stoically ignored finally became too much.

I can still see Dick sitting on the exam table during that first consultation: shirt off, looking as solid as a rock, but with tiny beads of sweat formed on his upper lip and forehead. There was a palpable mass filling the entire lower abdomen on the left. It was big, and hard, and sensitive when touched. Dick winced but only conceded, "That's a little tender there," when I pressed my fingers around its edges. When I examined the final segment of his rectum it was still soft, but at the tip of my finger I touched a stone-like mass. With endoscopy we were able to biopsy and confirm that he had colon cancer. A barium enema showed how tightly the tumor mass had constricted the distal bowel. Further x-ray studies indicated that fortunately his kidneys had not become blocked and still functioned.

At the time of surgery I went for a cure in the sense of doing everything I could to eradicate the malignancy. That meant not only a radical removal of the left half of the colon, but taking all the tissue off the major blood vessels and muscles that lay on its back side deep to the tumor. Up front the tumor had grown into the muscle of the abdominal wall. This is unusual but explained why the mass was there and why it caused so much pain. A portion of these muscles had to be cut away along with the tumor mass. Fortunately the rectal area was clear. I was able to bring across the right side of the colon and attach it to the last couple of inches of rectal stump so normal bowel continuity could be maintained. This was hard work; that day it was my turn to sweat.

Uncomplaining as ever during recovery, Dick soon returned to work. Not long after he left construction and took a day job as a city building inspector. This was an ideal position for him. He really did know everything about construction and had too much integrity to let anything substandard pass his inspection. For a time word got out in that suburban city that all construction now was subject to a higher level of scrutiny. Shoddy work was not permissible. That's the kind of reputation Dick had. With such an advanced cancer Dick probably should not have lived very long, but he went on for several years. For a long while there was no evidence of any malignancy and he returned to a normal life.

This had been a challenging surgical case but the real story for me began in those after years. Dick and I became friends. I was raising my family in a rural setting on a 28 acre farm. Doing outside work was what I did to decompress from surgical practice. I always had projects I was dreaming up but usually did not have time to complete them. Dick wanted to help. He recognized that my ambitious plans for building, remodeling, laying cable and pipe, were not supported by any experience. He came in for checkups periodically. I'd tell him about my latest project. He was just a great guy to talk to. Sometimes I would stop by his house on the way home. I liked to go there because he kept everything he owned so orderly and clean. Sometimes he dropped by my place in the country when he was out driving around. So for a number of years we had a wonderful relationship.

I insisted upon paying him when he did work for me, of course, but this was one of those arrangements where wise advice and help at critical moments went beyond any monetary valuation. In one poignant moment I remember, I was resisting, saying to Dick he was doing too much work for me and not charging enough. Dick put down the tools he was using and stepped close, standing directly in front of me. "Doc, I want to do this," he said, "I owe you; you saved my life." So we didn't talk about that again. For several years afterwards there was still no sign of return of his colon cancer. Dick got promoted to a higher supervisory job and we began to see each other less frequently.

Then Dick started having pain in his back. He thought he pulled a muscle on the job. He put off making an appointment but finally returned to see his family physician to have it checked out. He had x-rays and blood tests done and was told everything was OK. He tried the muscle relaxants and pain pills he was given and returned to work. I didn't hear about this until Dick called me weeks later. It was March, I think. He asked if I would personally review the x-rays his physician had been taking in the office. The backache persisted. Maybe I could figure it out. Maybe he knew.

That same afternoon I did go over to the family physician's office and looked at the films. I happened to spot one of those rare circumstances which lead to a classic oversight. It's one of those things they give you in training as a test so you won't get the idea you're too smart. There, behind disease-free lungs, the stubby twelfth rib on the left side was missing. The bone had been eaten away by a late metastasis from his colon tumor.

The rest of Dick's story can be distilled because the next months were not good ones and you can probably anticipate the outcome. The return of his colon cancer in this unusual way was confirmed by biopsy. It also involved the adjacent vertebrae. He was ultimately transferred to a Seattle hospital for intensive radiation and chemotherapy. All this stretched into the summer and then the fall. Along with Dick's very supportive wife and children, I visited him while he was there. There wasn't much for me to say. I kept coming but felt awkward. I could neither do anything nor think of anything encouraging to say. Dick faced all this with his usual stoicism. He was a man's man in every good sense and not likely to make much of what he was enduring. He didn't see any reason to discuss what he could see as the outcome.

When the end was near treatment was suspended. Dick asked to be transferred back to our local hospital which spared his wife a daily commute into the city center. His room in our suburban hospital was like a sanctuary of calm. His wife took to coming over in the evening, sliding into his bed just to snuggle up again with the man she had slept next to for so many years. No one on the ward said anything about this cohabitation. It was looked upon as a private matter that did not concern the staff. Every shift of nurses came to regard Dick as such a great guy they wanted to do things for him. Through the fall months Dick grew weaker and more emaciated. He still faced all his difficulties with such resolve and strength that the nurses came to admire him as I did.

I still remember the call summoning me one afternoon over the PA system. It was just before the Christmas holidays. Dick's nurse had me paged. When I called back she spoke to me with a wavering voice, "Dick's going. You'd better come." I wasn't far away and hastened up the stairs for what was our last visit. The nurse stood at the door, waiting to usher me in. As I entered she moved away and returned to her desk across the hall. That gave me a moment of quiet stillness at the bedside before family started to arrive.

My wife and I went to the memorial service in Dick's local church. The building was way too small. The community responded with a huge outpouring of respect for this every day sort of man. All the pews were uncomfortably packed. Mourners crowded around the walls and squeezed together in the narthex. It was a cold rainy day but a hundred more spilled out across the church yard and into the street beyond. A number of attendees rose to speak about what Dick had meant to them. That day a lump in my throat was burning too much for me to say anything. I had never attended a funeral for a patient before--always too busy, too busy. But from that time on I tried to attend every memorial service for any patient or

Renewal member. And eventually I did find my voice, as I am trying to do in writing this book.

I kept turning it over and over, "What more could I have done?" I knew in this case there was nothing. In our quiet conversations during those last months Dick had probably been more supportive of me than anything I did for him. Still, I knew there must be some way to stick closer with my patients, not be just the one who operated on them. After my encounter with Bernie Siegel and this experience with Dick, I decided to give doing something different a try.

That first letter I sent out does not exist any more. Keeping a copy never occurred to me. I was always very meticulous about details in surgery, but in things like correspondence I tend to be informal and spontaneous. Exactly what the invitation to my patients said, I don't remember. It went something like, "I was your surgeon. I am looking for some way to be more available to provide the latest information and answer questions, etc., etc.," Something fairly stiff like that. I do remember we made enough copies for the three dozen patients I selected from my list. I hand-addressed the envelopes and put them in the mail myself. I was a bit surprised that almost everyone invited showed up. It was January, 1982. There was no thought at the beginning of how long we would meet. We didn't know exactly what we would do, or where this would all lead. When I remember that first stilted invitation I am reminded of a quip I heard about the same time: People don't care what you know...they just know if you care.

The first meetings we held after office hours in the waiting room of my clinic. The space was packed. The situation caused awkwardness too if my partners had late appointments and were still seeing patients. Soon I arranged to use a small meeting room at the hospital across the street. We later moved from after hours time back to 4:00 pm so people could get home for dinner, but we stayed with meeting on Mondays. There was some experimentation. For a while we met in a section of the hospital cafeteria, for instance. And no time was perfect, but these were small matters. We discussed options for meeting in the group. We made compromises. Though there was some uncertainty with such a novel idea, the fact that everyone had some prior association with me helped a great deal with getting to agreement.

Beyond these arrangements there were only two philosophical points I thought important to explain to the group. First, I saw the meetings as something I wanted to do. I saw this as an extra service for my patients, a gift. As such there was never any consideration of charging for attendance. The second point I announced to everyone was that the concept was to be one of information sharing. It was to be an educational forum with give and take from all of us.

Up to this time I had not learned any differently. I assumed that I could just continue to talk about what I knew and others would want to listen. I could talk about diseases and treatment, offer up advice about diet and exercise, give health tips that helped minimize effects of certain illnesses. I planned to add current thinking about treatment of various types of cancer and answer technical questions about surgical procedures and their consequences.

I was wrong about this. What I gradually found was that there was, yes, a great deal of interest in what I thought we should talk about. And yes, respect for me as a physician helped move the conversation along. But mostly people wanted to have a chance to talk. They wanted to talk about themselves and their problems. They wanted to ask questions. As they grew confident in the safety of our meetings, individuals began to talk about very personal things. And if there was someone in the group with an experience similar to their own, a person might just as soon listen to that one as to me.

—m—

As I began Renewal I knew I needed help. I approached a clinical psychologist whom I knew. I admired this man in part for his wholesome sense of humor. He wasn't weird or creepy in a way that I knew would turn people off. He didn't go overboard with analysis. He turned out to be my faithful partner in getting the group started in the early years and provided a good balance. I was coming at this from the point of view of education as someone with experience in cancer care, but I did not have any real experience in counseling or complicated psychological problems.

So while I was still thinking through what this would all look like, I went to my psychologist friend and told him of my idea. Remember, again, support groups were virtually unknown thirty years ago, at least in our area. I was very pleased when he said he would not only be available, he would partner with me in making this happen. "Sounds like fun," he responded. So he and I together founded the group that subsequently became Renewal. I would not want to dilute in any way saying that without his help, Renewal would not have come into being or have been as meaningful.

For one thing, my friend was more skillful than I in complex psychological entanglements. He was able to maneuver around any hint of manipulation or any control issues that arose. An occasional new person would join the group and start running the same psychological ploys they employed everywhere else to manipulate others. In Renewal this was picked apart with gentle humor and kindness, not confrontation. The reward in this for the new member was finding, in the quickest way possible, that cancer had changed the rules. They as the disease host were still playing their life-long game which always worked up until now. As a cancer patient they needed to change. Renewal helped move such a person on to a more successful attitude toward their illness.

My psychologist friend was very skilled but also congenial and warm. He had a wonderful laugh that seemed to disarm any tense situation. He recognized that his sense of humor was an asset. "I got that from my mother," he said recalling her influence. "She would always pick up what was said and fire it back with some humor. Mother liked to laugh. I came to realize humor is important in healing. So, when I'm giving a talk, or when I meet with the Renewal group, I like to start by telling a joke."

I keep saying, He. My friend's name is Luke. Luke also said, "We cannot know what is going on in the head of a group member by talking at them. We have to get outside our intellect and listen."

About ten years after our meetings started Luke moved away. He closed his clinical practice and moved on to other things. He now does health and nutritional counseling with his partner Jess Aldin. Their website is www.healthyfoodhappylife.com. Because of what he is doing now, and feeling strongly about the importance of nutrition, he rather spontaneously recommended Michael Pollan's book, *The Omnivore's Dilemma* (Penguin Press, 2006), so I pass that along to you. Luke chose not to be identified fully in this story, but we did get together as I was working on the book and had a long conversation. He is very supportive of my getting the Renewal story out. He was as kind and open as he had always been and responded when I asked him for his recollections of Renewal and what had impressed him about the group. Here is some of what he said:

"I always saw this as a way for me to give something back," he began. "Some people thought their doctors were saying their cancer was their own fault, and that isn't correct. We had to tell people to stand up for themselves. I know people were very appreciative; they felt better at the end of our meetings.

"I always felt humble when I went to the Renewal meeting and in working with the people there. This was partly because you and I actually didn't know what those individuals were thinking. We had to either ask, or find out in some other way. We were helpful in healing, making the disease process more manageable."

He remembered some people in particular and called them by name, even though it had been years since he had seen them. Some of them are in Chapters 2 and 3 so I'll not repeat that now. "I remember Tom. He was good-natured, but sort of sour. We had to encourage him to stay involved because of his on-going pain and depression. We were helpful in healing or at least making symptoms more manageable. The outside speakers on things like nutrition were a help."

Luke remembered a young man named Chuck who had lung cancer in his twenties and had one lung removed. Chuck always wore cowboy boots. "You could feel the anxiety or pressure. He always talked like he was angry about something. Chuck had refused group therapy elsewhere but said he kept coming to Renewal 'to help you other people.' He was trying to deal with his own fear. I remember some others who were desperate and near panic when they first arrived."

I asked, what do you think is the value of a group such as ours?

Luke answered, "When somebody died, the group was powerful in how they helped one another. There was a grown daughter who came along just to help her mother get to the meetings. We encouraged the family members to attend, and to keep on coming after the cancer patient died, when they could. If you can get people to feel strong enough, and that they have the right to say what they want and don't want, they will make progress. We were never closed to what anybody said. The group could pick and choose what it wanted, like inviting special speakers. Some of the people who were speakers worked for the hospital, like the woman who taught a series on Tai Chi. Those hospital employees got to explore and advance some of their personal interests because of the opportunity with Renewal."

Luke had something he taught us about simplifying transactional analysis. It was a shortcut to actually undergoing analysis. There are three ego states: The first is to act like a parent. You say and do things your parents did, often without realizing. An example at work would be you tell a subordinate, "You will work the Christmas holiday."

The second ego state is acting like a child. You feel and act as you did when you were a child. You often got hurt, were afraid, excited, and sometimes hateful. As a child you have no power. An example at work would be complaining in response to the order above, "You never take your turn!"

The third ego state is to act like an adult. You deal with facts, deal with the present situation and make decisions without excessive emotion. For instance in this workplace example you might avoid conflict by saying, "There are four major holidays. They need to be split up evenly and then rotated. Which one do you want to take first?" So first decide if you want to use adult behavior or not.

How can psychology as a discipline help a person with cancer? Luke said, "First, it can help with depression. It clearly can get a patient and their family both to communicate and reach acceptance. The family, not just the patient, may have suppressed feelings and that needs to come out. There can be hidden resentment. Anger can build. If we can talk about those feelings, it may free up the patient to be healthier—if they can be relieved of that tension. For a family that is dysfunctional one person in the family may be 'the problem.' That label keeps the rest of the family from uniting to deal with everything else. Psychology can help people learn to support each other. And, in a dynamic group like Renewal, there can be cross fertilization. It's an educational process for everyone involved. In a group like ours, an individual is more likely to try something new, like having fun, because group support backs them up."

Drawing from experiences he had elsewhere as a psychologist, Luke added, "It's sort of like treating alcoholics. The worst time can be when they first stop drinking. The family may say, 'I liked you better when you were drunk!' Some people are ready to change. Maybe it takes something like cancer to get that change started. And once it starts, change or growth can be destabilizing to the family unit and its status quo."

During those years Luke and I sometimes conducted meetings jointly. Sometimes it was just one of us. Luke had this wonderful technique of relaxation. I recalled this, saying sometimes I could hardly wait for the latter part of a meeting; the sharing part would die down, and Luke would end things by leading us in a relaxation exercise. "Relaxation is important," Luke still agrees. "It can have a real impact on stress and how the patient handles, or mishandles, stress. You can do this without saying, 'This stress is why you got cancer.' Psychology has documented that relaxation techniques are good. Other scientific disciplines have documented reduction in stress hormones and the beneficial increase of other substances like endorphins."

Relaxation exercises help you to let go of tension. The technique Luke commonly used had us close our eyes and get comfortable. He'd have us descend on an escalator while he counted to ten. Then we could visit in our mind some safe and beautiful place like a Pacific Island beach or a secluded forest glen. After we had been there for a while, relaxed and breathing rhythmically, Luke brought us gently back into our meeting room by ascending the same escalator. He counted backwards from ten to one, similar to the way we entered our relaxation. After such an exercise we would all sit quietly for several moments, feeling like we actually had left the room and gone somewhere--some place where just a short time there helped us regain our energy.

From techniques of guided imagery you can branch out to letting the participants meet themselves as the child they once were. Let them develop a comfort with that. Have people bring pictures from childhood and talk about life as that child. Ask the person about their life as an adult and to comment, comparing then with now. This is different from dream work. Other techniques available to someone with experience are the use of drawing in various ways. Drawing can be used to express feelings about the illness. Automatic writing is another approach.

"The advantage of relaxation exercises," Luke concluded, "is that you almost instantly feel better. And, you can carry such a technique with you anywhere and use it at any time."

I usually wore a shirt and tie but it was not uncommon for me to come to meetings wearing a scrub suit. If I had been up all night I might be as pale or gaunt or disheveled as the most distressed person in the room. In those years I frequently worked to the point of exhaustion and really could sleep standing up. At such times, as the murmur of conversational voices continued, or we were having guided imagery, my head would slump forward and I drifted off for a few minutes, breathing loudly. No one ever said I snored, but maybe... In Renewal I usually played it cool when I awoke from an unintended nap, looking around like maybe I had just blinked and rubbed my eyes. I took a little ribbing about this, but the bigger thing was that the relationship we formed allowed the momentum of the conversations to move ahead unimpeded. This was one indication to me of the strength the group had developed. I had begun the transition from instigator/leader to being more of a participant.

In all our years we never established any rules of conduct. We all just showed up and began. We welcomed new attendees first, letting them pass if they did not want to speak. Then we went on to cover reports on a week's worth of activity from our members. These ranged all the way from people uncertain about embarking on a course of therapy to those presently undergoing treatment. Those who saw themselves as recovered might want just to talk about common daily activities. When the meetings broke up, we put away the various items we used or displayed and went home. This routine was sometimes displaced by a celebration or memorial service. Sometimes we went on field trips.

We printed a simple trifold brochure to explain ourselves to prospective members. One woman had an artist friend who did an ink drawing for the front page—it is the same picture that is on the cover and frontispiece of this book. My daughter Yvonne is a graphic artist and put the brochure together for us, just as she has done some of the art work in this book. Someone brought in their favorite quote to include in what we were preparing. We called it "A final thought." It's a nice one by Joseph Epstein and is included here for you to think about:

> We do not choose to be born. We do not choose our parents. We do not choose our historical epoch, or the country of our birth, or the immediate circumstances of our upbringing. We do not, most of us, choose to die; nor do we choose the time or conditions of our death. But within all this realm of choicelessness, we do choose how we shall live: courageously or in cowardice, honorable or dishonorably, with purpose or adrift. We decide what is important and what is trivial in life. We decide that what makes us significant is either what we do or what we refuse to do. But no matter how indifferent the universe may be to our choices and decisions, these choices and decisions are ours to make. We decide. We choose. And as we decide and choose, so are our lives formed.

Gradually I grew in my understanding of what we had started and what was taking place. I found that the participants wanted so much more than just the medical information I assumed to be paramount. We held our meetings to the time frame and schedule we established, but personal friendships grew. Relationships flourished outside our meeting times. All of us have holes in our personalities and our array of relationships. It would be wonderful if every cancer patient had a knowledgeable and fully supportive family and group of friends. Obviously that is not the case, even though quite a few members came to Renewal with a spouse, other relative or a friend.

Here is one of the central truths that made Renewal work: people came to Renewal because of self interest. It's part of mental health. Everyone intended to get what they wanted out of coming and we helped them clarify that intention. Some people drove quite a distance, some had to leave work early, and some put aside obligations at home in order to make the meetings. For many there was some element of sacrifice; maybe that can be equated with paying for admission or paying dues.

Most of us have an innate curiosity. When we hear about activity in someone else's life we want to listen in. We compare what we hear about them to our own lives. Our ongoing conversations in Renewal kept things lively. Even something as mundane as having the flu for a few days makes us wish for someone to take care of us. We regress a little. The mutual support in Renewal meetings gave people permission to do that for a time if they wished, but then they had to start moving forward again to keep up with the group.

The opening of this chapter might suggest to you that we are heavy into confession, analysis, and psychotherapy. That is not the case. We are much more animated, more into seizing the moment, and into supporting one another in difficult circumstances.

In no particular order I want to relate what were the important components of the success of our group. The most vivid memory of Renewal among all the people who have come, and there have been hundreds, is the parties. The gaiety, the reprieve from the grinding humdrum of being sick, was the energy of our celebrations. This tradition started modestly and grew over the years. It became the extracurricular thing we talked about the most. We'd recall the last celebration until almost the time to start planning for the next one. We started with common interest in having a potluck meal for Thanksgiving. The sentiment was one of thanksgiving and appreciation for what we had developed together as a group and we wanted to show it. Then came time for Christmas, New Year's, Valentine's, St. Patrick's Day, and the Fourth of July. New Year's parties included setting expectations for the coming year, a mind-expanding thought for anyone not so sure they would live another year. This came to include a candle lighting ceremony in remembrance of anyone who died during the previous year. For others lighting a candle could be a moment to recognize someone who had a special impact upon their personal outlook. We also held a monthly acknowledgement of all the recent birthdays.

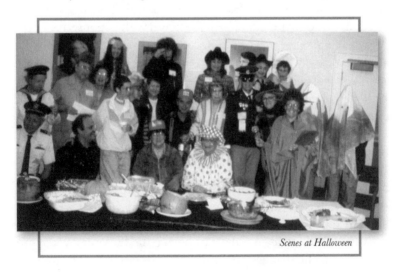

Scenes at Halloween

What came to be the biggest of all was...Halloween! Newcomers might hold back and do nothing other than wear a hat or something else modest. For established members it was a time to plan some expression of themselves. They tried to shock or amaze their Renewal friends and vie for the most original costume. The atmosphere was something akin to Mardi Gras in New Orleans. Unlike Mardi Gras it was a celebration for setting aside a period of trial and discipline, not approaching the start of one.

Another break in the routine of discussion at meetings was a regular cycle of guest speakers. This was doubly good for me. I could avoid speaking on subjects about which I had only superficial knowledge. I also could avoid appearing to advocate some concept that was on the fringe of medical practice or, maybe, completely outside it. When the group wanted a certain person, or to hear about some new concept, I used my medical connections to locate and invite appropriate speakers. Some who came were practicing physicians with a special interest like complementary med-

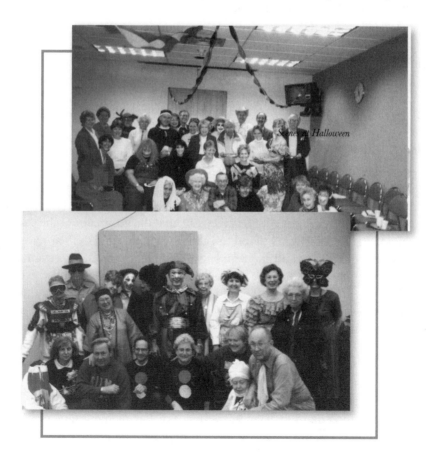

Scenes at Halloween

icine, but not all. There were some instances where speakers came at the invitation of a group member. Such visitors responded to the wide breadth of interest in our group. A rare one made baseless assertions or had a commercial interest in promoting a product, usually some dietary supplement. The group proved very tolerant of such pronouncements but was unerring in identifying bogus claims. I became quite proud and confident about the sophistication of our members.

My physician colleagues occasionally asked if I weren't afraid of exposing some vulnerable person to radical ideas. I knew I was under some scrutiny and was quick to say how mentally healthy the group's outlook was about novel suggestions. And, well, the truth is, members hungered for new ideas. Many had gone as far as conventional medicine could take them. Some had rejected the edict, "There's nothing more we can do for you" from their physicians. For some Renewal members their personal experience in treatment had been unfortunate. Their situation and/or personality had been matched with the wrong advisor or the wrong treatment.

Talking about diet and exercise is commonplace nowadays. Making changes in such matters and sticking with them is not easy even with considerable motivation. In Renewal we were able to break down some resistance to change with actual demonstrations. Some were kinesthetic or experiential adventures for the group. With diet we studied changes to prevent cancer long before that idea became the popular news item it is today. We explored whether what we eat might augment conventional therapy. We periodically had daylong seminars, usually at someone's house, where we could have demonstrations and cook.

Our first and most lively proponent of these ideas was Ms. Virginia Brown. Virginia lived on the opposite end of the state but welcomed invitations to come and meet with us. She educated the group about the value of bio-energetic food (that is, food substances that are close to their natural state and have not had all their nutritive value leached out. An example is comparing the food value of sprouted nuts and grains to commercial crackers we purchase in cardboard boxes. The latter have no nutritional value besides supplying empty calories). Virginia was an advocate of the vegetarianism advocated in the 1940s by Professor Edmond Szekely of Rancho La Puerto in Mexico. She also advocated an interesting approach to positive thinking. She said whenever we realize we are having a negative thought, say, Cancel! to yourself and substitute something positive.

When the book *Recalled by Life* by Dr. Anthony Sattilaro came out in 1982, recounting that physician's experience of having metastatic prostate cancer, Renewal went through a cycle of studying macrobiotic diets. This has the concept that includes eating only certain types of healthy food in season, and eating only foods grown near where we live. One of our dearest men in the group was an indefatigable supporter of his wife in her treatment of breast cancer. Though he worked full time he took over the duty of doing all the cooking for the household so his spouse could follow the macrobiotic diet she wanted.

Our study of Ayruvedic medicine was legitimized when it was presented to the group by a local M.D. who was well established as a conventional practitioner. About as far out as we ever got was to experiment with the growing of kombucha mushrooms. Actually kombucha, or kobucha as it is referred to in parts of Japan, is not a mushroom but a type of lichen that grows to look like a giant mushroom. The root word in Japanese, kobu, means kelp, as in seaweed. There is quite a process ritual in maintaining these growths. We decanted the broth from its lichen parent and drank it as a tea. It's certainly more dramatic and involved than buying kombucha capsules at a health food store. Participating in growing, preserving, and processing food as Renewal did captures the attention. It gets people involved. It helps create an appreciation of nutritional value. Like many of our undertakings as a group, this kombucha ritual was accompanied with a great deal of mirth. Some took the assignment of maintaining our private stock, sort of like maintaining sourdough starter, and hauling it to the meetings. Some would partake of the cold tea and some did not. There was a healthy attitude supported by the group that it didn't do any harm to try something new—and it might do some good.

The conversations around this tea drinking offered yet another opportunity. It gave encouragement to individuals to share what they had experienced or heard about in ingesting all sorts of nostrums. When we had potluck meals their variety provided an opportunity for people really into dietary changes to educate others. This succeeded not only on the level of demonstrating cooking skills but also became a manifestation of a member's dual commitment to change and to helping others. This same attitude of adventure carried over into what members shared as they worked out for themselves what to do about exercise programs or how to reduce stress.

—m—

When we started I had no idea how powerful symbolism was to a person's life. Over the years Renewal kept adding symbols to our group culture. These became the basis for creating the traditions that made our group so distinctive. It caused our culture to be strong. The most frequently used of these symbols were from Native American tribal customs. One of these was our talking stick. Our particular talking stick was a gift brought to us by a guest speaker, Dr. Michael Murphy. It was carved by a member of one of the Northwest coastal tribes. At the meeting where he presented the talking stick Dr. Murphy showed us how he had learned to use it and make it part of his family meetings.

Thereafter, following his instructions, we passed the stick around our circle, letting each person in succession hold it. The holder had permission to speak whatever was foremost and true for them at the moment. If a person wished they could choose not to speak and pass the talking stick on without comment. This passing of the talking stick continued until no one in the circle had anything more to say and the miniature wooden totem passed a complete circle in nothing but silence. This process was a powerful inducement. Even newcomers or the most shy tended to join in. Holding the stick was implicitly a moment of empowerment; you had permission to speak and an attentive audience. It became the holder's chance to share their concerns in a safe environment.

The second most influential symbol for us was a gourd container from a separate Indian tribe. After having its purpose explained to us by the Native American healer who presented it, we adopted a tradition of filling the gourd with our New Year's resolutions. It became our vehicle to the future among a group usually ensnared in present entanglements. This was much more than an empty gesture for Renewal members. Every member carried his or her own concerns about cancer treatment, the possibility of recurrence, and family matters. The gourd and our New Year's resolutions were a time to put on paper an ambition or expectation for the coming year. These notes we marked with a personal identifier. Usually at the first meeting of a new year we brought the previous year's notes out again. This offered a moment for comment on what our intention had been when we wrote a year earlier. Then we could either embrace that as a continuing wish for a subsequent year or choose to refine our hopes with something new.

As you might expect, sometimes it was left for a surviving spouse or other caregiver to retrieve such a note from the bowl after its author had died. The emotion and candidness expressed in such revelations proved for some to be achievement and happy memories. For others reading a resolution was cause to express disappointment. Always it was a way to move along any grieving process. For some there was growth, for others rededication.

At least twice a year we would have the candle lighting ceremony. We kept and used candles in various colors and sizes. The variety allowed the one choosing a candle to recall a member lost to the group, a way to highlight a trait of that individual's personality. We kept a shallow clay bowl for holding the lighted candles. Inside was a mixture of sands and rocks. It was our custom to have anyone who made a trip bring back a bit of sand, small rock, or shell from some far away place. The new item memorialized that journey. That trip's significance to the member was transferred to the clay bowl. We always dimmed the lights before beginning our ceremony and used only natural light from the bank of outside windows. This was one of several ways we honored members who had died.

Lighting a candle could also be an occasion to say something encouraging to a member still alive, perhaps even present. This ceremony could take a long time because of the thoughts and emotions members wanted to express. By the conclusion our bowl was ablaze with the combined light of many candles. The flickering light surrounded by semi-darkness seemed especially bright because of the remembrances that had been spoken as each candle was lit. And, only twice did we set off the building's smoke alarm!

We accumulated quite an assortment of other relics to display. Most came as contributions from our members or were left with us by guest speakers. It is amazing how we look differently at a rock after we hear someone tell a story of where it had been discovered at some special moment. We had bundles of tobacco, bones, herbs and trinkets used in Indian

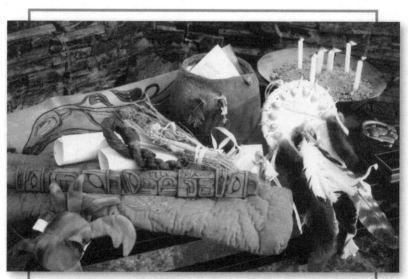

Some of the symbols from Renewal traditions: Talking stick and embroidered sheath; gourd with New Year's wishes; tobacco and sage for smudging with other items from Native American ceremonies; otter totem; dream-catcher; candle dish for memorial ceremonies.

smudging ceremonies. There were various utensils some guest would have used to perform a cleansing ritual. We had a hand-carved sacred otter totem, a dream-catcher, a protective shield of Indian feathers and shells brought by a Medicine Man from still another local tribe. It helped us that, when Dr. Carl Simonton talked to the group, he mentioned some of his experiences while being invited to participate in sweat lodge ceremonies with tribes of the Great Plains. Some of these physical symbols still exist and are shown on the previous page.

Another mainstay of the group was our lending library. Renewal started as an educational group with the books from my office. Over the years members brought in a wide range of books and tapes they used. Others we bought. The only money which changed hands was what we collected periodically by passing a tin cup. We used donations for books, refreshment supplies, and to subsidize the parties. Some of the people with medical backgrounds supplied volumes with technical information. Some members felt buying books was an unnecessary expense. Others had just never formed a habit of reading much of anything. For them it was very meaningful to have someone put a book into their hands just as a meeting ended and say, "This has helped me a lot; you need to read it." What was being offered might be a copy of one of Dr. Siegel's books like *Love Medicine and Miracles*, or Dr. Carl Simonton's *Getting Well Again*, or anything else on diet or spirituality, or maybe something germane to that day's discussion. It was the personal recommendation coming from one member to another with the book that made the difference.

Over the years we collected photographs of almost everyone who came to the meetings. These we added to collages and framed. Most meetings they were put up and displayed around the room. This gave each

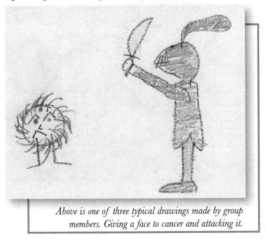

Above is one of three typical drawings made by group members. Giving a face to cancer and attacking it.

individual a sense of belonging and confirmed equality seeing their picture with all the others.

We had special songs, poems, and stories composed for us. Somewhere between physical symbols, rituals, and subjective experiences we were introduced to the value of music. We had several wonderful speakers over the years who provided analyses of why great composers have been able to affect us with the sound of their work. These speakers partitioned the various types of music into that which would soothe us and that which would stimulate and fortify us. They helped educate us in how to make selections and use such knowledge to help ourselves. In a similar way we periodically repeated courses of instruction in Tai Chi, yoga, and simple stretching exercises to harmonize our bodies. We had instruction on how to use art and drawing in various exercises to get in touch with our inner wisdom.

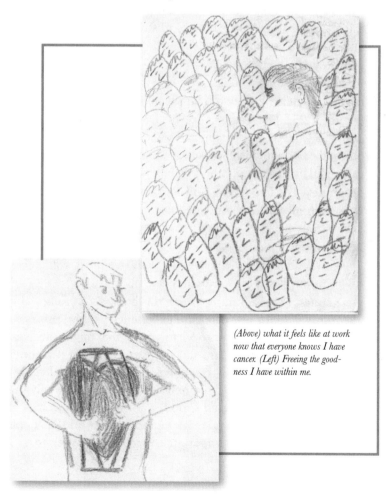

(Above) what it feels like at work now that everyone knows I have cancer. (Left) Freeing the goodness I have within me.

Ten years into these meetings I felt a desire to summarize some of what we collectively had learned during our first decade. I still have that announcement sheet and have copied it below. It is sort of an interim summary as we continue on through this book and prepare to hear individual stories. These topics were well founded in our group experience. As we began a new year I used these six topics for quick review and a general discussion. It may help you to think about each subject and relate it your own experience. The six subjects I chose to cover in the initial meetings of that particular year were these:

January 4: The Key to the Lock: Forgiveness. Unless a cancer patient jettisons all injustices of the past with forgiveness the burden is heavy. The door leading to any new path remains locked.

January 11: Relaxation, Meditation, and Visualization. Each is a separate, powerful tool in strengthening the body and returning to health.

January 18: Amplifying Powers of Visualization with Neurolinguistic Programming. (This one is still valid but probably too esoteric a diversion for purposes of this book.)

January 25: The Importance of Diet and Supplements. Some of what we have eaten and some of what we deprived our bodies of both have weakened us. Proper nutrition helps us defend against illness and regain health.

February 1: Maintaining and Regaining Health with Exercise. Strength, flexibility, endurance, and confidence all derive from exercise. Start with a basic program of walking.

February 8: Finding What's in Us: The Use of Drawing. This is one method to get in touch with our inner self and discover our own true desires and destiny.

My two greatest reservations in writing this book about Renewal were how to relay the essence of our collective experience without simply reciting case histories in a linear way, or to tell too much that might cause someone personal embarrassment. I also did not want to evoke memories of times and events effectively laid to rest. In researching the book I contacted a number of old members for their comments. I received only encouragement to tell their stories. They said it not only was all right to use their names for authenticity (there are no made-up stories here, only a couple of forgotten names), they felt it was important to record this experience. *They wanted their stories to be told.*

Some people, when we talked about this, took the additional step and wrote their experiences themselves. Many expressed the hope we could use what happened to them to help someone else. So as I have begun to do, I will introduce you to Renewal members. As you read on I hope you can make some association with a person's story. I assure you that person was, or still is, a real individual from our group. Use of first names maintains a degree of privacy, but to those from Renewal who read this, first names will be enough to evoke a clear memory of someone important to all of us.

So this book is some of our stories and experiences. We share among ourselves in group meetings and now share with you. Many of our members learn to progress from ignorance and confusion, occasionally from shame, embarrassment, or desperation, to something better. In Renewal we have been rewarded many times by seeing a member, still contending with matters related to his or her own disease, express a desire to reveal their personal saga. In such a moment this sharing elevates the rest of us and takes us beyond preoccupation with self.

If you have cancer yourself, you still may be at the early stage of coming to terms with your diagnosis. You may feel simultaneously both fear and anger. Maybe you are asking the common questions, "How did this happen to me?" And, "What did I do wrong?"

When I hear someone say, "I am a cancer victim," my first reaction is, that is an unfortunate way to see yourself. Something has happened and something presently is. That does not necessarily make you a victim. From the minute you get a diagnosis established you need to choose a positive viewpoint. Put yourself in charge. Devise a strategy to be the victor, not the victim. So, throughout this book we avoid victim and minimize using even the term patient. Renewal is not a doctor's office or hospital. Renewal is not in the business of making diagnoses or dispensing medication. Renewal is about self-awareness, commitment, accountability, and collaboration. We often emphasize whom we are trying to reach by using the term "your self" instead of the conventional "yourself." In preparing this book we have tried not to get into the mode of writing a doctor's prescription. We minimize saying what you need to do and try to avoid being formulaic. Read what is here and learn for your self.

No problem for a Renewal participant was so severe it could not change to something better. Simple words and candidness have the power to connect us with others. Truthfulness and openness can unveil a disease process and reveal sudden insights. Collecting our experiences and sharing them with readers is the collective contribution of Renewal members. We are ready now to draw you in. We want to make you effectively a participant in our meetings. How you use the experience and how valuable it becomes will depend upon how much you decide to do for your self. "My cancer may kill me," one woman at Renewal blurted out spontaneously, "but it has given me back my life!"

Some thing, or some one, brought you to this book. Perhaps in your mind everything about your health is OK. Or conceivably, you see this as the worst moment in your entire life. Anyone can create desire and determination and acquire new knowledge. You may be exploring to learn more about your illness. Reading this book suggests already you have avoided the denial that paralyzes when too much bad news comes too fast. You may reach a new place where you ask, "If that's my problem, where or what is the solution?" Next comes asking, "What can I do to help myself?"

Renewal welcomes such people. It is a place to query others and explore your self. We acted upon the proposition that Yes is the answer. In your realm of motivation consider carefully, "What is my question?"

On the journey of serious illness there is always a time of being alone. One of the wonders of our group is that parallel experiences began to converge. Bringing our separateness together provided an opportunity for synthesis. We learned to speak in a context of healing, understanding that healing is not synonymous with cure. Cure as understood by the average person sometimes comes, sometimes it does not. We found a new and unexpected power to heal even in the absence of cure. That is a central message of this book.

Meeting with Renewal for almost 30 years changed me. I'm glad to have been there. I hope after reading about us you will feel changed, and glad too. The grace and love evident in the stories that follow is a kind of truth, like a gift ready to be presented. Both grace and love are inside you now, waiting. As you read along, when that gift reveals itself, we hope you are open to accepting it.

This chapter opened with an excerpt from a poem written by my friend David Whyte. The title is "Everything is Waiting for You" in a book of poetry by the same name. Here the poem is in its entirety:

> *Your great mistake is to act the drama*
> *as if you were alone. As if life*
> *were a progressive and cunning crime*
> *with no witness to the tiny hidden*
> *transgressions. To feel abandoned is to deny*
> *the intimacy of your surroundings. Surely,*

The Meetings

even you, at times, have felt the grand array;
the swelling presence, and the chorus, crowding
out your solo voice. You must note
the way the soap dish enables you,
or the window latch grants you freedom.
Alertness is the hidden discipline of familiarity.
The stairs are your mentor of things
to come, the doors have always been there
to frighten you and invite you,
and the tiny speaker in the phone
is your dream-ladder to divinity.

Put down the weight of your aloneness and ease into
the conversation. The kettle is singing
even as it pours you a drink, the cooking pots
have left their arrogant aloofness and
seen the good in you at last. All the birds
and creatures of the world are unutterably
themselves. Everything is waiting for you.

CHAPTER 2

THE MEMBERS ———————

"In the middle of the road of my life I awoke in the dark wood
where the true way was wholly lost..."
— *La Commedia Divina*
Dante Alighieri (1265-1321)

"Every saint and genius has told us two things: we are not guilty of error nor
called on to correct it; and the plan of life is built into us and
its truth can never be removed."
— *The Bond of Power, Joseph Chilton Pearce*

In this chapter we begin to explore stories of individual members of the Renewal
group. We will look at some of the problems that arose and how they were resolved. Some
experiences I recall and others come from interviews. We use actual first names; it is the
member's way of leaving a personal mark: this is my story, what happened to me. As
Renewal went along we were too much in the moment to think of recording our activities
for the long term. Fortunately many members are still alive and able to talk about those
days. Their recollections reveal our central theme.

— Joan —

Joan is a woman who shows how the course of a cancer can become
very complicated. It can affect the course of an entire family unit. Joan
was 36 in 1990 when she was diagnosed with breast cancer. She knew
even before that about her aunt who had prepared for a career as an opera
singer only to die of metastatic breast cancer at age 41. In later years Joan
felt guilty that she, who also followed a career in music as a professional
violinist with the Seattle symphony, had lived but this aunt had not.

Joan actually was found to have cancer in both breasts. The left breast
had a less common tissue type which was already Stage 3, while the tumor
in the right breast was an infiltrating ductal carcinoma, Stage 1. She re-

members the tumors being described to her as golf ball size on the left and the size of a grape on the right.

It is significant here that a cousin, a woman close to Joan, had been diagnosed with breast cancer about six months prior to Joan's surgery. This cousin, Kim, was only 28. Although Kim was told her tumor was Stage 1, she quickly developed signs of metastases. Both women came to Renewal together a few times, but Kim soon became too weak to continue.

By the time Joan had her diagnosis she saw how much the lymph node dissection and perhaps repeated chemotherapy injections had made her cousin's arm swell. Joan, knowing such an occurrence would end her career as a violinist, refused to have node dissection. She remembers reviewing the operative permit just outside the surgery suite and discovering that it stated "with node dissection." She refused to sign and made the staff call her surgeon in for personal assurance that this was not going to be done no matter what the paperwork said.

In both biopsies the margins on the tumors removed were considered inadequate. Joan was told to have a second, more extensive excision on both breasts. She was very upset about this and consulted two other surgeons for advice. She was told in both instances that these things happen and that the repeat operations were indicated. So two more procedures were done. After recovery a course of radiation treatment was devised. The areas radiated included both breasts, underarm areas, and the base of her neck. One complication of all this was that Joan's singing voice suffered. She lost her voice completely for a time but even when she could talk again, singing as a considerable source of pleasure never returned.

Joan was anxious and distrustful concerning her radiation. She explains it like this: "As a trained musician, I am very sensitive to pitch in sound. After a few treatments I could tell that sometimes the machine "hummed" in a different way, at a higher pitch. When I asked about the difference in the sound and said, 'You must have given me the wrong dose,' the technician denied it. But when I made them check, they discovered that they had left the setting on what had been used for the last patient. I can also count time very accurately. So I could count, 1…2…up to 45 seconds when the radiation dose was supposed to end. Once it went on for a minute and 45 seconds! When I complained, they realized a mistake had been made [and a compensatory skip in the treatment regimen took place] and another adjustment had to be made."

A Groshong catheter was placed as an aid for adminstration of chemotherapy. This semi-permanent, indwelling device meant her infusions and blood draws could come out of a large central vein without any discomfort. Joan thus avoided any trouble with her arms becoming swollen. She kept the catheter in for ten months. Still, the additive effects of chemo were disabling. Each time she had an infusion of her combined therapy she would lose her balance. Her husband would generally have to help her walk back to their car. "Also," she adds, "I would be mentally conked out for eight or nine hours. This is when I discovered by talking to another Renewal group member that Coenzyme Q10 would help me. Taking Q10 made the mental side effects much better. I was functional again in just two or three hours after my infusion."

It was during this dark time that she started attending Renewal. "I tried several other groups, but they were too depressing." At Renewal she met others she could identify with, notably another woman from the Seattle symphony, and began to read and talk to others about how to have a better quality survival. She got her questions answered and appreciated the nascent humor, even when it was somewhat macabre. "I remember one time a man who had to wear a catheter and urine bag made a joke about himself," she recalls, "It was really pretty gross, but it was so unexpected that it made everyone, including me, laugh. Then I realized it had been nine months since I had laughed, and then I really started to laugh!" After that she checked out books and humor tapes from our library.

"I got really close to the core group of members," Joan remembers. "One man in particular talked to me and gave me courage. He had melanoma, and was dealing with recurrence and having a hard time of it, but he still helped me and others. He and I talked both inside and outside the

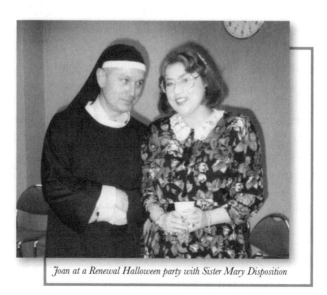

Joan at a Renewal Halloween party with Sister Mary Disposition

group meetings." [A short time later this man shot and killed himself.] "That just broke my heart."

Joan also had a sister who developed breast cancer. The sister has survived for many years, but recently had a recurrence. Their mother, Alice, had multiple myeloma, another type of malignancy, and also came to the Renewal meetings several times with Joan.

"I got so much good information," Joan adds, "When you're feeling hopeless, anything helps. Most doctors and nurses don't understand when you try to tell them how restless and uncomfortable you are; how the injections make you feel all prickly, or make your head hurt, or your mouth dry. There was always someone at Renewal you could talk to who knew exactly what you were talking about. All these things helped. And, after I started reading, I experimented with all sort of things: supplements, potions, all sorts of things."

During these months Joan grew ever closer to her cousin Kim. They shared the hardships of their treatment. Joan was holding her own, but Kim kept getting worse. Even though Kim's initial assessment was Stage 1, metastases had shown up early and her disease progressed rapidly despite very aggressive treatment. Joan could not separate herself from the observation that both she and her cousin had been diagnosed as Stage 1, with the implication of excellent prognosis, and it had come to this. Before her first year was out, Kim developed both spinal and brain metastases. For a while the two were able to continue to commiserate and share even after Kim was hospitalized. At one such visit at the hospital Kim told Joan she had a dream the night before. Part of the dream Joan remembers was Kim telling her, "The angels came to the window." Kim paused to raise her arms in a gesture in that direction, "Then they came in and got me to take me Home."

Shortly thereafter Kim lapsed into a coma. She was already bedridden in the hospital and for over three days had been totally unable to move. She died in the hospital, momentarily alone. The nurse who came in and found Kim reported to Joan and the rest of the family that somehow Kim had gotten out of bed, unassisted. She was found lying against the wall, her arms upheld toward the window.

Joan grieved about this loss and all the family's troubles, but slowly recovered. After a year's absence, she returned to her chair in the symphony. She continued to play until 2002 when she took a fall and injured her wrist in such a way that she could not continue to perform at peak levels and had to retire. Her husband also retired and the two of them chose to leave the city and move to the Camano Island near Seattle. "We live in a log cabin in the woods," as Joan now describes it. Joan has taken college courses and prepared herself for another career, unwilling to stop working entirely. At present she commutes a short distance to where she works at a state park.

— Margaret P. —

Margaret P. by coincidence also is a professional violinist. When I called her about this book the first thing she said was, "And on August 15 I'll be 17 years old!" That didn't immediately register with me for we hadn't had a conversation in years. Later Margaret clarified that she had just celebrated her 61st birthday in conventional terms. She went on to explain her present point of view is that her cancer diagnosis, the treatment that followed, and the successful outcome of all that were the beginning of a new life. She arranges things around that pivotal time as being part of a new start, a new birth. But where she came from, and what happened, were not easy.

In 1989 at age 43, Margaret started having what she thought were hot flashes from menopause. When she kept getting worse her physician did some blood work. The tests that followed indicated that she had chronic myelogenous leukemia (CML).

She is quite open in discussing how she thinks she got there. "In 1989 I was very low," Margaret told me, "My husband had left me for someone else. I was raising two teenage children. I had no money. I was trying to hold things together by playing the violin and giving music lessons. Prior to the diagnosis I had pretty much given up on life. When I found out I had this cancer, my first reaction was that I had found my socially acceptable way to die."

She was told her diagnosis in a telephone call from her doctor on the Wednesday before Thanksgiving weekend, 1989. The first specialists she saw after that told her there were no treatments that would cure her. She should expect to die in three to five years. When it was explained to her that the mutation of a chromosome called "Philadelphia" was the genesis of this malignancy, her interpretation was that she had caused, or allowed, this mutation to happen because she had given up on living.

Then she was referred to the Swedish Hospital Tumor Institute in Seattle. There she met a young physician, Dr. Richards, who was doing a fellowship. "He told me there was another way," Margaret remembers. "He told me about bone marrow transplants. This series of conversations is what started the nine months of deliberations, the 'Do I or Don't I?'" She refers to these nine months as her gestation that occurred before the rebirth with her transplant. It was a long nine months with many considerations.

One consideration was money. She was told that a bone marrow transplant was going to cost $10,000 up front before the institution would commit. Even before that $2000 more out of pocket would be necessary to pay for tissue typing. Friends helped raise money for her care. Bone marrow transplants had been successfully pioneered in Seattle but at that time were still classed by insurance carriers as experimental. Fortunately, just three months before her procedure, Margaret got the good news that the AMA had taken a stance that validated the value of these transplants. Still to come was another imbroglio with her insurance company. She had changed coverage to a new company a short time before the diagnosis. The new insurer took the position that this was a pre-existing condition. "They refused to believe I didn't already know I had cancer," she remembers. With the help of a lawyer she got that straightened out and obtained the coverage she needed.

Then there was the risk. Her chances of success, of living, were 48% based upon statistics at that time. Her age was beyond what was considered ideal. Margaret remembers thinking there was nothing she could do about that. She was advised that a certain number of people undergoing this procedure could suddenly grow worse for any of a variety of reasons. If such complications did occur, there was about a 30% chance that she would just die suddenly.

Still another problem adding to her deliberations was the lack of a donor match for replacement bone marrow. No one in her family was a match. The U.S. donor registry had no match. Then, what she recalls as one of the steps along the path of commitment, she asked for them to check the European registry. This was still during the time when everything was being done on Margaret's dime and this decision carried significant additional cost. Then, on Valentine's Day 1990, she got a call. There were eight perfect matches for her tissue type in Europe! Ultimately a man who is still unknown to her was chosen. All she ever learned about him was, at that time, he was a resident of Amsterdam.

All this investigation filled the nine months. Was it worth the gamble? She had to accept that death was a likely outcome. Having no assurance of survival meant Margaret had to consider her son and daughter, 18 and 19 at the time. She was told with the transplant she could live several years or die suddenly. Without the transplant she knew she would die, just more slowly. That was the choice she weighed. She remembers a clear choice to come down on the side of life. She decided that her family, her love of music, the feeling that there was more for her to do in life, all weighed in the balance tipping her to take the chance on the transplant.

Margaret started coming to the Renewal meetings in January. Renewal played a part, but Margaret did the hard work on her own. She felt that emotional well-being was a key. She had to reach a place where she knew that even if she lost this gamble, if she died, she was not a failure. This meant, of necessity, letting go of so many things she had come to believe made her sick. She had to unburden herself of a lot of baggage. She started reading voraciously. One of her first books was Dr. Bernie Siegel's *Love, Medicine and Miracles.* Another book she found extremely helpful was something that had also just come out, *Flow,* by Mihaly Csikszentmihaly (Harper & Row, 1990). The author had interviewed Auschwitz survivors, among others, as a resource for the book. She accepted as true that author's conclusions about his own research. Briefly stated, to her it was, if you look back on the time in your life which is most memorable, about which you have the most pride, it turns out to be when you had to stretch and do something you never thought possible. You did something you thought you would never be able to do. Margaret recalls that she didn't even finish reading the entire book. With this explanation she had gotten the inspiration she needed. "I intended to live, but I had to feel that *there was nothing else* I could have done to help myself."

Margaret correctly remembers that there was little published material available at that time, little access to audiotapes, etc. This is one of the ways the Renewal group helped her. She sums up these several months as being a time when she felt she needed to make her body as pure as possible. She gave up alcohol, caffeine, sugar, anything she felt weakened her body. She drank lots of water to flush her system. She designed her own fitness program and exercised as much as possible. "I developed a runner's heart," she remembers, "I had never been in such good shape in my life." She took supplements. She took herbs. She drank herbal tonics by the case. The tonics were delivered to her from a source in New Mexico (she thinks). She sought out a psychic who lived in another state as an independent advisor. She and this woman talked every week. After a time the psychic was delivering messages: she could "read" Margaret's body as a mosaic and gave interpretations of what was going on inside. "You tell the doctors to look here and to do this or that…" she directed over the phone. And Margaret delivered those messages to her care givers; she no longer cared what they, or anyone else thought.

Margaret reported to the hospital feeling in top form for all the extensive preparation that was to follow, but still carrying the knowledge that her chances were a little less than 50%. As the treatment killed her cancer it also destroyed her bone marrow and all her immune defenses. In those days this destruction led to sterility precautions and isolation in a laminar air flow "room" where no one could approach her. Such reverse isolation is no longer practiced. It was found later not to affect survival. Her daughter was Margaret's mainstay during this period. The daughter compiled a contemporaneous notebook of pictures, quotes, and loving messages to bring to the hospital. This sustained Margaret during these long weeks when no one could touch her except in some clinical way. Margaret saved her daughter's album all these years. She got it out when we visited and shared the pictures below. The first picture is from that very day she remembers as her lowest ebb in treatment. "That's it," she handed me the first picture below, "That day was the worst."

August 15, 1990, was the day of the transplant. That was the day of "rebirth" and how Margaret has stylized all subsequent events. Everything

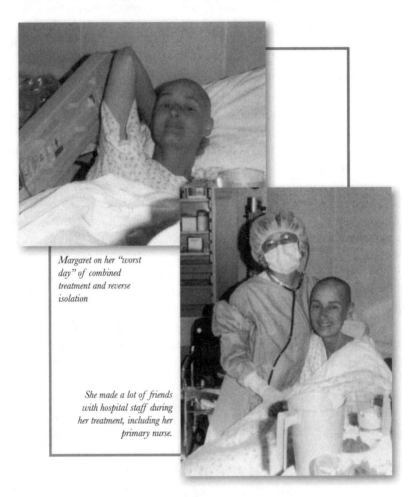

Margaret on her "worst day" of combined treatment and reverse isolation

She made a lot of friends with hospital staff during her treatment, including her primary nurse.

else aside, she demonstrated remarkable composure and awareness to have formed so many new friends during this difficult time. During rehabilitation after the transplant she and her physical therapist became friends. They made a promise to each other to climb Mt. Rainier south of Seattle if Margaret survived. So exactly one year later, to celebrate this first birthday, the two of them trekked as high as they could up Mt. Rainier and had their picture taken. Margaret made a similar pact with her daughter Erin who spent much time with her. The two of them made a pact. If Margaret pulled through they would celebrate her five-year survival when it happened. The two of them promised to make a pilgrimage to Amsterdam to honor the donor of the bone marrow. The donor had specified he wanted to remain anonymous. Margaret wrote the man a letter but never found out if it was delivered. So five years later, after receiving medical clearance that she was "cured", she and Erin traveled to Amsterdam to be there on August 15. They went to celebrate both this fifth birthday and a milestone

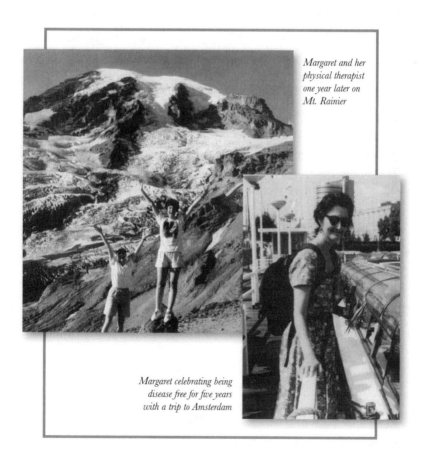

*Margaret and her
physical therapist
one year later on
Mt. Rainier*

*Margaret celebrating being
disease free for five years
with a trip to Amsterdam*

in a new life. There was no one to visit and thank in person, but it was an important symbolic gesture to Margaret.

There were complications after the transplant. For one thing, Margaret got shingles (herpes zoster) that sent her back to the hospital for another form of isolation—into a room with a steel door, she remembers. While there she got some clarity: "I had this dream about opening a conservatory to teach young musicians," she recalls. She had been considering this as a life's goal off and on for twelve years before she became sick. After she recovered, Margaret founded, and still directs, the Seattle Conservatory of Music. She sees her work as providing instruction to young violinists who want to become professionals. She travels all over the world as an extension of this vocation.

Margaret gave back to the institution where she received her treatment. From about 1991 to 1994 she frequently was called upon to come to the hospital and share her experience with people undergoing bone marrow transplants. She also gave speeches, wrote for hospital publications, and helped with fund-raising. Finally, she went back to her music and being Margaret. She participates in music institutes internationally. The day after we talked in 2007 she hurried off to spend a summer teaching at an institute on the East Coast. A trip to China was in the planning stage.

As her fiftieth birthday approached Margaret decided to take two months off from work, even though it wasn't her best economic decision. "I was 50. I looked at it as half my life was behind me and half still ahead." She chuckled, dismissing living to 100 as not necessarily an important goal. "But it was a good moment to enjoy, then decide on something else I had been wanting to do. So I went to England.

"For two weeks I stayed in London. When I first went south I stayed at Amberley Castle. They gave me Queen Elizabeth's room, even though they weren't supposed to. When I walked to Stonehenge I could see it in the distance. I walked the bridal path; someone there told me I was walking the path of the great King Barrows. Then I went from Devon through Cornwall. When I was in Cornwall I had the sense I was traveling in an ancient land—it was beyond old. I found that every church was built on a pagan site. I stayed in hostels at first. Then for six weeks I walked and stayed in all sorts of places. I took the Southwest Coastal Path around Land's End. Five hundred miles on foot." She separated what she was saying for emphasis, "Alone. With a backpack."

She took a ferry to the Scilly Isles. "I talked with people about their ancestors, about the times when people could sense more." She paused to look at me, "Did you know that when the fog came in, those ancient fishermen along the Cornish coast could sense their way back home? Same with travelers on foot, they could sense their way to where they wanted to go. It's the lay lines, they call them. Just like migrating birds find directions. It's the magnetic lines and the old people could sense them."

On the coastal path each day she looked out at the sky and sea meeting on the horizon. She wrote in her journal, took pictures, and pressed flowers. She went on, "I felt at peace. I came back a new person. I had spiritual experiences the whole time." Then she stopped. She turned and looked at me anew, smiling, "Not all who wander are lost."

Margaret sees clearly that she got to do these things only because she persevered and she lived. During her time at Renewal she formed a friendship with Gary, the same man Joan mentioned in her story at the beginning of this chapter. Gary was the man who was having a very difficult time contending with a recurrence of melanoma. Still he found a way to participate fully in the group and not only explain his problem but help others. While Margaret was in isolation during the transplant Gary called her and sent letters frequently. She thought he was everything a friend should be. Then, while still in isolation, she got the word that Gary had shot and killed himself. "I got very angry at him," Margaret remembers. "How could you do this?" she still asks the question with emotion, "How could you give up? I was really mad. I needed him!"

Margaret's story has gone on to quite a level of detail. I did so hoping to help the reader realize how tough this was for her and then see the rewards that came after. The suffering was real, but so was the transformation. I highlight this to prepare you for something else Margaret told me. There is one more aspect of Margaret's success story to share.

Her closest friend at the Renewal meetings was a woman working through her own separate issues with breast cancer. She too had difficult decisions to make. Aside from their friendship this was someone else who helped form Margaret's conclusions about this entire experience. "She and I spent a lot of time together outside the Renewal meetings, talking," Margaret told me. "We got to be such good friends that I invited her to attend a workshop with me. It was a program on Therapeutic Touch, a method of laying on of hands to help someone's ailments. It was a really special event being taught by the originator of the technique, Dora Kunz. Dora must have been 93 or 94 at the time, really old, but amazing in what she did and in her perceptions. Dora was also clairvoyant."

This friend of Margaret's in Renewal was a cornerstone of the group. She was held in high esteem by all of us. Margaret paused for a moment in our conversation. "After the Therapeutic Touch conference, as we were filing out of the room, Dora Kunz spoke to me about my friend. Dora pulled me to the side and said, 'She isn't going to make it—your friend—she isn't going to make it.'"

Then Margaret paused again, punctuating this, "I got where I could do the same thing." Then she continued, "All those years, talking to people at the cancer center, I got where I could tell who was going to make it. I'd hear later about this one who made it and that one who didn't." Reading the reaction on my face, she added, "My nurse friend is the same way. She's the one who went to Amsterdam with me. She told me she could tell too. After a while she left the transplant service. She works somewhere else now." After still another pause, Margaret concluded, "It's a presence. Some people have it and some don't."

Margaret looks back now and believes that some people are stronger than others. "Books and all that help. They are amazing but *you have to apply what you learn!* It takes hope, but it also takes action! It's action in every way: physical, like everyone saw me doing, but it's also mental and emotional. I had to work on parts of me nobody saw. I had to heal relationships; I had things about my childhood to take care of. There are things I'm still working on. It's part of the reason I'm going to New Hampshire tomorrow. There's something else that still needs to be taken care of. I believe we are all born with certain issues in our family, problems we have to solve. If we live, we have an opportunity to solve them. There is no question that I would not be alive without the expertise of western medicine. But there is also no question that my survival was enhanced, maybe depended upon, embracing holistic medicine and in my dealing with the emotional aspects of my illness." Margaret started walking me to her door. As we parted, we agreed to keep in touch.

Margaret has a joy, a passion. She has created, by her own industriousness, a novel way to have one of the great passions of her life, teaching young musicians. When I checked in with her in 2008 Margaret told me, in addition to having her own school in Seattle, she was Scholar in Residence at the University of Colorado. She started juggling going to Boulder two days a week, "I'll be teaching music teachers how to teach." She concluded by saying, "I have the most wonderful life now. Every year gets better. And now I get to spend time with my grandchildren!"

As I left her house Margaret came out onto her front porch. We had spent much of the afternoon talking but the sun still shined brightly. She called after me, having just thought of one more thing to say: "You can tell the ones who will live. Those who are not willing to do everything to get well just want to negotiate about their illness."

— Jane —

Jane is another woman who made the very writing of this book rewarding. I had to make some inquiries but finally tracked her down a few months after starting this manuscript. I finally obtained a phone number and just called one day to ask for her story. I said hello and gave her my name. I thought Jane might well have forgotten me after so much time had passed. Then I quickly went on to ask, might I interview her for inclusion in the book? What did she think now about the whole experience with cancer?

Jane chuckled before she said anything. This response caught me off guard. "I've been waiting for 20 years to tell you what I think." She laughed again, "What you told me in Renewal changed my whole life."

So, let's back up for a minute and give you more of the story before we get to that part.

In 1987 Jane was 45 years old. She was an associate in the most prominent law firm in our area. She had been busy at work and finally had a mammogram after three years of procrastination. She was told she had an area that needed biopsy, but not that her mammogram showed an almost certain breast cancer. She saw a local surgeon and had the lump removed. She was told it was cancer. Then she was told the excision was not complete. The margins were not clear. Jane remembers how upset she was that somehow in those initial conversations no one told that she probably had breast cancer.

She came to see me as a patient. At that time a plastic surgeon and I had started a clinical trial of doing a combined mastectomy, when indicated (that was my part), along with an immediate reconstruction (that was the plastic surgeon's part). This was a novel approach when we started this about 1980. I was pleased with our results and suggested to Jane this was a good option for her. Jane still remembers the date. "It was September 10th," she told me. "I was told after the procedure that the nodes were negative for metastasis, but despite the good news I was still depressed for the rest of the year."

Unfortunately it was only a few months later, in January, that Jane noticed lumps under her arm. We removed them the next week and they proved to be cancer in residual lymph nodes. At that point Jane agreed with a recommendation she have chemotherapy. It turned out to be a bad experience. Jane was aware that during this same time period I had operated on the wife of one of her law firm's partners for breast cancer (a woman who has done well and never had a recurrence) and that I had also seen one of their paralegals. The paralegal was years younger but had a large and rapidly growing breast cancer. She had tried chemotherapy but had not tolerated it. She refused any surgical treatment and died within a few months. This paralegal was a friend of Jane's and seeing her die was demoralizing.

It was about this time in early 1988 that Jane started coming to Renewal. She was still working full time at the law firm. At this point Jane digressed in her story to relate something about the individuals she remembered from the meetings. In particular she remembered a woman who was eating so many carrots to increase her beta-carotene intake that the palms of her hands turned orange. She also remembered being impressed by a woman guest speaker who talked about interpretation of dreams. "Then," Jane returned to addressing my questions on the phone, "You told us a story that changed my life."

I had no idea what she was talking about, but she cleared that up as she went on. "You came to one of those Monday meetings and told us about one of your old patients. You had seen him over the past weekend. I remember you were pretty excited. You told us he had been a Boeing engineer. About ten years before you had operated on him for cancer of the pancreas. [It's a big operation called a "Whipple" for a cancer that has one of the worst prognoses. Only about five per cent of patients with the disease used to live five years.] "You said that you had not seen him in all those years and assumed he was dead. Then, the previous Saturday, you and your family were walking down the street in the University District when you saw him. He was older but you recognized him immediately and he recognized you. You told him how pleased you were to see him and asked how he was doing."

Jane is still telling me this over the phone. I am silent because I don't remember any of this. And, I still don't know where this is going. "He told you he was fine," Jane continued. "He'd never been back to see you or any other doctor. When you asked him what he had done to stay healthy, you said he told you he had taken your advice. He reminded you that after this big operation he had come back for follow up a few times—he had some tubes in his stomach, or something. At some point he asked, what he should do now? He quoted you as saying, 'There's nothing more to do. *Just go out and live your life.*'

"So he told you, still standing there on University Avenue, that's what he had done. First he quit his job at Boeing because he didn't like it. Then he went back to his home in north Seattle and became a gardener. He had always loved gardening. Growing flowers was what he enjoyed more than anything else and it was what he really wanted to do. After a while people in his neighborhood started hiring him to put in flower gardens for them. That's how he made his living now."

Jane switched back to talking about herself, "I heard you say that and all of a sudden I knew what I wanted to do. I went home that night and thought it over some more. I needed to quit what I was doing. I didn't like my job either. If I ever wanted to realize my dream of living on Whidbey Island and have a garden, I had to move there as soon as possible. I'd have to figure out a way to make a living in that small community. I asked my family to meet with me. I needed to ask their support and forgiveness, for doing what I wanted meant I could not continue to support my children financially while they were in college. It was the hardest thing I ever had to do, to tell my kids I couldn't help them anymore. I wanted their forgiveness. The kids were great.

"The next morning I went back to the office, asked for a meeting with one of my partners and told him my decision. They were relieved to get rid of me. I had not been pulling my weight at work recently and they feared a lawsuit if they dumped me while I was ill. Smart folks. I stayed long enough to turn my cases over to other lawyers in the firm. I left in about a month.

"I had always wanted to have a garden too," Jane connected back to the man from Boeing. "And I wanted to live in the San Juan Islands. I wanted to go out and live my life. If I were to survive, fine. If not, I still wanted to be doing what I wanted where I wanted."

So Jane moved to Whidbey Island. She began working for another lawyer there. It was too far from her new home, so she left and started her own solo law practice. She had designed a house and had it built, and became a gardener. She has continued in that practice until the present time—but on her own terms. She told me she has related this story about the changing direction of her life to many people over the years.

She went on to tell me that not everything had been easy just because she did that. For one thing, getting health insurance after she quit was a major problem. She qualified for Cobra coverage for six months, but after that all insurers wanted to exclude breast cancer from her coverage. With all the other changes, it was a scary time and she felt vulnerable. She and her first husband had divorced before all this happened, so she faced most of these challenges alone.

Fortunately Jane had a long-term loving partner whom she married in 1990 so she could get health insurance. He came to Renewal with her for a time. He encouraged her to continue because he liked the group. "He was so impressed a physician and a psychologist were leading it."

Jane explored dream interpretation and read everything she could get her hands on. Oliver Sachs (author of *The Man Who Mistook His Wife for a Hat)* became one of her favorite authors. She explored her spiritual side with the Whidbey Institute (www.whidbeyinstitute.org). She taught free legal seminars twice a year and slowly has built her law practice. She focuses on estate planning and elder law, drawing on her teaching experience and medical knowledge.

Jane took up kayaking on Whidbey. Through her practice she met two women who started wilderness adventures of various sorts, including annual kayaking, under the name PeerSpirit (www.PeerSpirit.org).

Exasperated she was not getting satisfactory answers to many of her medical questions, Jane did research on breast cancer in the University of Washington Medical School Library. She sat in the same carrel where she had once studied for zoology exams as an undergraduate. There was the frustration of dealing with multiple institutions and doctor offices so Jane started keeping her own personal medical record. It was a tedious fight, but she finally got every health facility to copy and send all their reports directly to her. After that she brought her records with her to medical appointments so she could negotiate for more careful management of her case.

At Swedish hospital she berated the Quality Control office long enough to get her records released. She took to reading all the nurses' notes from her records, feeling they gave her the best understanding of what had taken place. She continues her own research on breast cancer. She decided to take the hormone-blocker Nolvadex and did so for almost eight years. She got a lot of information from the University of Washington after she started going there. She started using her computer and www.mymedical-records.com. as a resource. Jane is ahead of her time on this. She wishes every patient had a portal into their medical records no matter where the records are generated. The medical community still is resistant.

She had to have a gynecological procedure done. Based upon unusual sensitivity to sedation (blood pressure drops, heart rate slowing) she insisted upon a personal meeting with the anesthesiologist assigned to her case. She remembers he didn't like this inconvenience at all, but came around after she explained herself. They talked for 45 minutes. With this preparation, she did not have any trouble with this anesthesia. Afterwards she sent the anesthesiologist a box of chocolates. They are on good terms now.

All this openness and spontaneity in telling me her story impressed me. I was even more impressed a few days later in speaking to Jane's legal assistant to find out that at the time we first talked Jane was less than a week away from having yet another surgery. Periodic follow-up had revealed a spot on one lung. After a needle biopsy had confirmed this was a new cancer, she was slated to have this second malignancy removed. Later I asked Jane about this. Her answer implied having this lung surgery wasn't a big thing. She had been down this road before. Whatever was to be would be. She hadn't mentioned it in our first conversation because, well, I hadn't asked!

Jane had the lung tumor removed by the new minimalist techniques done in the chest nowadays, similar to laparoscopy done in the abdomen. The lung tumor was malignant, a non-small cell cancer as it is called histologically, and the procedure was a complete success. Within a few days Jane was back home again. When I checked in with her almost a year later, the middle of 2008 and again in 2009, she was well and had no signs of recurrence.

So Jane is back in her island home, doing what she has always wanted. She says she is living her dream. All these medical problems are a distraction, but she feels she has all the facts, knows how to deal with anything new that comes along, and is in control of the situation. And she has her garden. She issued a sincere invitation for me to come see it. She'd like to show me what she is so proud of—a life she has created for herself.

— Nancy K. —

This is both a story about one woman and her illness and a story of how one of our members moved beyond that period to have an effect on a great many people. Nancy recounted what follows in several telephone conversations we had. She was 47 years old in 1998 when she was diagnosed with inflammatory breast cancer.

Inflammatory breast cancer or IBC as Nancy refers to it, is a particularly aggressive form of breast cancer and usually ends in early death. Before her diagnosis Nancy had never heard of it. She remembers being both angry and sad at the same time when she got this news. Part of this anger was directed at the lack of information available. "Here I was being told I would probably die, and it was from something I never had heard of before," she told me. "Most women have heard the admonitions about investigating any breast lump they find on self-examination. Who has heard that some swelling and redness that looks like an infection or bug bite might be a kind of cancer?" Nancy has seen statistics that 70% of IBC cases are misdiagnosed at first. "I mean, I was always such a good girl, taking care of myself," she recalls, "Now I had this thing that was going to kill me?"

Fortunately Nancy consulted a good oncologist. This woman physician advised not to pay attention to anything Nancy might read if she researched the disease because, as she remembers, "All the books would tell me that I will die!"

Once Nancy and her doctor reached an agreement that they would go to the max to try to arrest the disease, they embarked on a very aggressive course of therapy. The first salvo was a combined regimen of chemotherapy: 5-FU, Cytoxin, and Adriamycin that was continued for six full courses of therapy. "My doctor told me she would give me the maximum dose of each drug every time," Nancy explains, "but she told me that before every session she would ask if I was too sick or weak, and if I wanted her to back off. I never once told her that...regardless of how I felt." After that Nancy had both a course of radiation therapy and a radical mastectomy. "When my breast was removed eight of the ten nodes were positive." Later in the therapy Nancy took Taxotere (synthetic taxol) followed by radiation on the affected side. She now takes Femara, an estrogen blocker. "I'll be on that the rest of my life, since my cancer was both estrogen and progesterone positive."

"I was so sick," Nancy recalls, "sometimes I would be vomiting once an hour." During such times she just moved into her bathroom at home as a practical matter. She took a blanket and her pillow so she could stay there. There were complications too, such as a serious blood clot caused by her Portacath that caused her entire left arm to swell.

One of the effects on the family was what Nancy feels she did to her daughter. This daughter, her only child, was 26 at the time. The daughter had an infant and was trying to establish her career. Nancy was trying to help by babysitting. Seeing her mother's suffering spooked the daughter. "My daughter was petrified. She was afraid what happened to me would happen to her. She actually considered having a bilateral mastectomy just to keep that from becoming a reality."

As these months of therapy dragged on Nancy reached one of those pivotal, life-altering moments. It's the time when a person realizes that things can't go on the way they are. Something must change. "I realized my family and I couldn't take this," Nancy told me. "I knew I couldn't do anything about the vomiting, (nothing had helped her aside from eating oatmeal or mashed potatoes), but I could do something about my constant crying. So, I told myself, I had to start thinking differently."

For starters Nancy tried to embrace the vomiting. "I made it a positive thing. I started to visualize that the chemo was killing the cancer and that was what made me sick—I was vomiting up the cancer cells. When Nancy lost her hair she took that as proof positive the Adriamycin was strong enough to kill the cancer too. "That shift made me feel I was in control," Nancy remembers, "and I would feel better—at least for three or four days until time for the next injection."

Nancy recalled how as a younger woman she had meditated quite regularly. She actually had done something like that off and on for thirty years. For a while she taught visualization at her church, taught teenagers how to use visualization to get along with their parents, for instance. When her child came along, and with all the duties associated with that, the times she spent looking inward became less frequent. Nancy decided to return to her old friend meditation during her year of treatment.

"I didn't know what an actual cancer cell looked like," she went on, "so I started to study about them, to learn more." She asked to see slides of her tumor's histology. "Then I started getting my own ideas. I'm what I call a 'realistic meditator'. I don't see cancer cells like some pretty white flowers in a field. To me cancer cells are like ugly, twisted knots tied in a black rope." She understood from her investigation that cancer cells can line up, move through tiny lymph ducts as they progress towards lymph nodes. "Later I began to visualize using my finger tips to pull those black knots or ribbons of cancer cells out through my nipple."

Nancy self-diagnosed herself as having "chemo brain." This condition has to do with the cognitive damage and induced memory loss that happens to people from the toxic effects of chemotherapy. Nancy is the first person I knew to pick up on these effects. Once she realized what was happening, she moved to counter these effects. "I challenged myself with computer puzzles, games—anything. I worked every day to make it better." She also recalls, "I went to a naturopath, I took supplements, I tried to eat better. I think changing my diet increased my energy level all by itself. I gave up red meat. I used no dairy, ate nothing white, and I drank lots of water to flush out my system. I also wanted to hear what worked for others and that is another way Renewal helped me."

A period of guilt emerged as Nancy's survival continued. "So many other wonderful women I met were dying. I wanted to be alive for a reason, not just because I was somehow lucky."

During this time of introspection another change began. Nancy told herself, "There must be a reason why God let someone with a mouth as big as mine live. God must want me to talk about this!" So she started talking to people about breast cancer, IBC in particular. "I talked to everybody— people I met in the line at the grocery store—anybody!"

Another one of her actions was to contact the federal government to find how they decide which research grants to fund. "The process involves

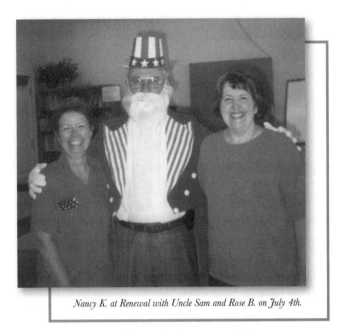

Nancy K. at Renewal with Uncle Sam and Rose B. on July 4th.

meetings of a panel of 20 research experts and three cancer survivors who critique proposals and regulate how federal grant money is spent. I thought, 'I'm a survivor, I've been through the terror of treatment for IBC. They need to hear from people like me.' I wanted to be sure the process was de-politicized."

Nancy ultimately was invited to participate in a three-day panel in Washington, D.C., sponsored by the Department of Defense Army Medical Breast Cancer Peer Review Panel. "I learned so much," Nancy recalls, "but I also told them, women with inflammatory breast cancer should be consulted. I asked them whether they knew enough about taxol? Did they know enough about side effects? At one point in this room full of Ph.D.s I stood up and said, 'I disagree with what you just said.' And they listened!"

Nancy went to dinner one evening with her scientific panel, including one of the researchers from George Washington University. "He asked me if I thought women would like to know about ways to improve their immune system. And, did I think women would want to know that being happy would improve their chances?" His research had convinced this scientist that stress hormones made the immune system less effective. "I asked those scientists why they didn't do something to promote support groups? They can be used to reduce stress and improve immune systems. They can be used to give us some hope and peace, even if it just lasts for a minute." She has continued to participate in this peer review process for the last six years.

Nancy has gone to a hospital close to her new home and started her own support group. She saw it as a group for developing coping skills with reliance upon meditation and the giving of emotional support. That experience has made it easier for her to tell others about what she had learned. The most recent time we talked Nancy told me, "I'm feeling great! I'm feeling strong!" She had just begun teaching a water aerobics class.

Nancy's passion about educating the public about IBC made her realize she had to get some type of media exposure. There was an IBC Foundation in the Seattle area and so she started attending their luncheons. "Everyone there was frustrated," Nancy remembers. At one of these luncheons she was given the name of Patti Bradfield. "Patti had a daughter of her own who was in her 30s, and had Stage 4 IBC." Patti previously had been an investigative reporter for the Seattle Times newspaper so she had connections. She desperately wanted to get the word out concerning IBC. It took a lot of convincing but the paper finally did a feature article on the subject of IBC. They interviewed Nancy.

Patti succeeded in getting the notice of a local ABC affiliate, KOMO TV. Their news department was persuaded to do an interview. Patti was so distraught about her own daughter that she felt she wouldn't be able to speak on camera without sobbing. "So she asked me to do it," Nancy recalls. "That news feature and the series that followed got on their website. It got 20 million hits." KOMO TV won an Emmy for those reports.

"We wanted to publicize the symptoms of inflammatory breast cancer. I had read that IBC is mis-diagnosed initially 70% of the time. Since it is usually diagnosed as a breast infection, or mastitis, and treated with antibiotics [partly because most of the women were so young] valuable time is lost. IBC is only six per cent of breast cancer, but it accounts for 25% of deaths. I've seen numbers that say survival is 40% after five years but only five per cent at ten years." Nancy changed the subject for a minute, "We lost a 16 year old girl to IBC a couple of years ago in California. At first the girl wouldn't tell her mother because she was too embarrassed. Then she was so young when she did see a doctor she got treated for a breast infection. By the time IBC was diagnosed correctly it was too late. The girl already had brain metastases and died within a few months.

"I am effective because my IBC was so bad," Nancy reflects. "Yet here I am, still alive and thriving. It will be my tenth anniversary coming up in a few months. I got over it with survival skills. That's what I talk about now, how to fight and survive."

During the years Nancy came to Renewal she was not only a member but a resource for us. She often led the entire group through one of the very visualizations she had created for her own use. Three of these are recorded in Appendix I. "You can't just suffer along in silence," Nancy concludes. "If I don't do anything my mind will take me to dark places. That's not healthy. It was best for me to shut that out by visualizing something positive. I don't care what image I use; visualizing helps me with a mental and emotional release. If I can get rid of my fear it helps me relax. Then I can go on and do something worthwhile."

— Bill —

Bill's story has a different kind of intensity. He exemplifies the Renewal member who would never give up. Sometimes that worked but in Bill's case even that was not enough. When I met him in 1980 Bill was a successful young businessman. He had a very close family. He was about thirty then and we had first met socially. I liked his way of living a good life. I think he thought it was prudent to know a few physicians he could count on and as much as said he wanted me on his list. Bill had a very strong alpha male personality. He was very self-confident, very interested in the pursuit of a succession of attractive young women. I heard he had finally found the right one and had gotten married.

Bill married in 1983. His wife recalls that despite a very strong constitution, he was not his normal self for nearly a year after the wedding. He went to see his private physician several times but was told his problem was he worked too hard. In early September of that year Bill felt feverish and went back to see his doctor. This time a blood test was done which showed that he was profoundly anemic. He got a call about this just before Labor Day weekend. After receiving some bad news he wanted to come see me. I talked to his regular physician then arranged to see him right away. The most prominent physical finding was a large mass in the lower right abdomen. Barium studies showed narrowing of the last segment of small bowel. This could be any of a number of things but all led to the conclusion that surgical exploration was necessary.

At the time I operated I found a large inflamed mass growing into and around the small intestine. It was attached to everything. I removed the entire obvious tumor and put things back together. Examination of the surgical specimen revealed this mass was a lymphocytic lymphoma, Stage IV because of the degree of involvement. Bill recovered uneventfully and took this bad news quite well. He felt it was a relief finally to know what his trouble was. By the time of discharge he had begun his own investigation.

He picked the best known medical oncology specialist in the city and we both agreed such a consultation was the best next step.

Bill's wife, Toby, remembers this time differently than I do. She recalls the anxiety leading up to this surgery, not knowing what the problem was, then getting the bad news that this was an advanced malignancy, and within three days also learning that she was pregnant with their first child. As soon as practical Bill was started on an aggressive course of chemotherapy under the direction of his oncologist. He and his wife agreed to the precaution of banking sperm samples, since the treatment would necessarily make him sterile. After their daughter was born the next year they used the banked semen for artificial insemination and later had a son.

One story about Bill set him apart from all the other members of Renewal for all time, and he frequently recounted it. After the chemo began his oncologist wanted to add a course of radiation to Bill's entire abdomen to try and sterilize any residual tumor. Bill agreed and the course of 30 doses began at a facility in Seattle. Bill said this process was pretty impersonal: put on a skimpy gown, lie on a cold slab of a table while some humungous machine centers over you with a whine. The staff scurries back behind a wall of shielding like a bunch of mice and leaves you alone. It was this last image that bothered Bill. Everyone acted like they were scared of something and left him alone to face whatever it was with practically no clothes on. Bill just lay there for long minutes while the technicians behind their shielding could be heard turning dials and flipping switches.

After the first couple of these treatments Bill decided to turn the tables on them. From that point on, every time the big machine began to hum, Bill would start to complain. He was being energized by the experience. He was…starting to have an erection! Some incredible energy was filling his body! He called out that his penis was getting impossibly big and began to moan as if the pleasure of his treatment was going to lead to an explosion. The therapists peered out through their portal. What was going on out there? The whole scene was counter-intuitive. The women especially could never get beyond their consternation witnessing this reaction. Bill got a huge kick out of the act he put on and schemed how to make it even more dramatic.

At first the combined treatment produced favorable results, but as the second year, and then the third, dragged on, the tumor kept growing back in Bill's abdomen. It became increasingly resistant to everything used to attack it. Bill's oncologist had established his reputation partly for his willingness to go beyond the bounds of conventional protocols. If the patient concurred he would devise one new regimen after another. After that came the experimental protocols and finally, true creativity.

This is where a second characteristic came into play for Bill. He was physically strong and withstood all this punishing therapy without complaint or loss of optimism. "Bill didn't ever give up," his wife Toby told me as she looked back on that time. "I think the really amazing thing is that he eventually did die."

While all this conventional treatment was going on, Bill got interested in what he could do for himself. Part of this came from his association with Renewal, but I will admit, once his search began, Bill went beyond anything I could have suggested. He was determined to overcome his disease and his financial situation allowed him to pursue any lead.

To tell this as a short version of the story, Bill tried to examine many of the alternative theories about the cause of cancer and investigate the treatments that followed as a consequence of them. He went to the Livingston Clinic in San Diego. He went to Mexico and visited a number of practitioners. He got literature from a cancer society in California. He heard about some doctor with an unusual philosophy in rural Washington State. He was on the East Coast; he was at an alternative cancer center in the Midwest. He found places I never heard of. Bill might call me at home in the evening to report he was somewhere out of state, checking out a new theory or philosophy about cancer treatment. What did I know, or what did I think, about this idea or that one? About the only influence I was able to exert during that time was that I didn't think it necessary to extend his search to Europe or the Far East. I reasoned with him probably he could check out almost any idea without having to leave our continent.

Beside this clinical side of the fight, Bill waged a war of understanding his own psyche and the psychology of being a cancer patient. He wrote longhand on plain typewriter paper because he wrote so much. He rambled over many things, then copied sheaves of these notes. He either mailed them to me or handed over packets at Renewal meetings. Some of these were about content at Renewal meetings. Some summarized seminars he attended. Some were introspective, just thoughts he conjured up by himself. I still have a lot of these notes—I'm looking at a stack of them as I write this. Bill struggled with self-diagnoses of being too negative and being too judgmental. He wrote about his innermost feelings while enduring chemotherapy. He wrote about how asking forgiveness was something to be analyzed completely then acted upon.

After a four-year fight Bill began to slowly slip away. All the while he remained aggressive and determined. He said he agreed he had a bad diagnosis but would not accept what others concluded was inevitable. Then he began to have internal bleeding and required blood transfusions. The cancer was displacing his bone marrow. "It was just one doctor visit after another," his wife told me. In the absence of much else to focus on, she remembers Bill obsessing about his platelet count. He had to be hospitalized. She remembers that in that last seven months of life he was able to come home only once.

"I was at the hospital with him every day from eight to five," Toby remembers. "It was just like having a job." She was now raising their two children like a single parent, alone except for the support of her parents and in-laws. "I told the kids later, when they were old enough to hear it, that if it hadn't been for them, I'd have driven my car off a bridge."

Even the oncologist, who would support a patient to any length, told Toby that in the beginning hope is OK, but now no protocol was going to cure Bill. At one of their treatment conferences he put before the two of them, "There is such a thing as false hope."

It was April when the last day came. Toby remembers, "Bill got up from his hospital bed, staggered and slipped right in front of me, falling over backwards. There was blood all over the place" And then he was gone.

Toby told me much of this, filling me in on these intervening years since Bill died. "I spent 14 years alone, just raising our two children." The older daughter has graduated now, their son is in college. Six years ago she found someone new and remarried. Then, with no apparent self-consciousness, added, "But I only changed my name last year."

— Bob H. —

Bob H. is an example of the type of person who came to Renewal with a sense of urgency. He was in real, acute distress. Most of the time Bob came to the meetings with his wife Jean. She came along because she was at her wit's end. Renewal really wasn't set up to function as a treatment center like an emergency room, but newcomers wouldn't know that. Bob and Jean came to their first meeting in 1995. Bob had surgery for cancer of the rectum in December, 1994, and started on a course of radiation therapy. In their first meeting the wife did all the talking. Bob just walked around the room.

Jean told the story of their life together. "Bob worked at Los Alamos on the atomic bomb," she spoke with obvious pride. Then, with more hesitation she explained some of the symptoms leading to Bob's diagnosis and his subsequent treatment experience.

While Jean talked Bob had said practically nothing. He just kept pacing up and back on one side of where we were all sitting. At first I thought he was just uneasy being in a room full of strangers. "Why don't you sit down and tell us what's going on?" I asked him. But he did neither.

Gradually over the next couple of meetings we found out Bob didn't sit down because he couldn't; he was too uncomfortable. Sitting down hurt too much. The radiation therapy had inflamed his pelvic area to the point of causing constant pain. It also created a general discomfort and anxiety that was hard for Bob to explain. His bladder also was irritated causing spasms and constant urgency to urinate. The medication prescribed brought no relief.

So Renewal got to know Bob H. mostly with him standing up. Progress showed itself in the weeks that followed the completion of his treatments and as inflammation gradually subsided. Bob was negative and cynical at first, but that began to change as he improved. Once he felt better, Bob turned out to be a really nice guy. Jean too was relieved as she saw this improvement and became happier and more relaxed. For the next year the two of them attended Renewal meetings faithfully and made a real contribution to our discussions.

The couple had to contend with another major setback in 1996. Their daughter was diagnosed with inflammatory breast cancer and died in a matter of months. The loss of their daughter weighed heavily on Bob. It was good then to have the group to support them. "There were a lot of good people there," Jean told me recently. "They helped us a lot." She reminded me she and Bob used to make trivets out of breadboards and contributed those when we had some occasion for gift sharing at Renewal.

After five years they gradually stopped coming. Bob just wanted to stay home and putter. "Bob spent a lot of time hand-building steam engines with our grandkids. He loved doing things like that with them. He also got to take the grandkids for a ride on a steam engine train. He got to take the son of our daughter, the one who died of the breast cancer, on a special trip like that. Other than those kinds of trips we stayed home and had a big garden. We got to celebrate our 60th wedding anniversary." Bob succeeded in overcoming a very difficult time during his cancer treatment and had another decade to be with his wife and family. He died in 2007 at the age of 84.

We had a second Bob, Bob L., who had prostate cancer. He eventually died from complications of that disease. He and his wife attended Renewal off and on for several years. He was a very quiet man who mostly enjoyed being at home. His major interest was collecting antique electric toasters.

Over time he educated us about how broad the interest is in collecting toasters in America. I bring this up because of the classy way this Bob planned his exit. The somber moment of his funeral turned to a lively occasion as we saw the good-natured humor in what he planned for himself. At his memorial service, which many Renewal members attended, the featured display was not flowers; it was his huge toaster collection. Funny how such a quirky personal thing can linger on as what we remember most.

We had yet another Bob, Bob A., who also had colon cancer. This third Bob came to the meetings for several years with his wife. He was a retired United Airlines pilot. He usually sat there, marking the interactions with his changing facial expressions, and letting his wife speak for the two of them. He would participate but gave the impression that being there was just a chore. He perceived Renewal as something necessary to stay healthy and prevent recurrence. He is still healthy. This Bob I remember so well because he made such a point of telling me that he didn't like me, at least not at first. Once we sent out a questionnaire to people who rarely came any more, asking what they remembered about coming to Renewal. Bob A. wrote back: "I didn't like Dr. DeShazo. He never would tell me what to do. Whenever I did ask him something like that, he'd always tell me that I needed to figure out what was best for me."

— Artie —

Artie is a woman whose story is a testament to how tough people can be. She was our poster girl, if you want to say that about someone who is old. She probably influenced more people with cancer at Renewal than anyone else. This was due in part to longevity; she came for 20 years, but she was always positive and upbeat despite her many troubles. Artie was also quick to confront the downheartedness many newcomers spilled out in relating their stories. The other reason people tend to think of her first when they think of Renewal is because of the difficulties cancer posed for her and her persistent optimism.

I first met Artie when I did her surgery for breast cancer. We had just started Renewal and I invited her to the meetings. What was so unusual was that over the next 15 years or so she had four more separate types of cancer. The second was a new malignancy in one lung. That was successfully removed. Then came colon and thyroid cancers. The final was in her nasopharynx, the back of her mouth. After this last malignancy was excised she had a course of radiation therapy to the mouth and neck that made life very hard. Her teeth had to be removed. Even after the pain of the treatment subsided, her tongue did not work normally. That in turn affected her speech. Artie could not swallow or eat well enough to sustain her and required a small feeding tube down her nose and into her stomach. Later this was replaced with a permanent feeding tube inserted directly through the abdominal wall. She had a lot of pain with these radiation treatments and was self-conscious about her articulation.

Artie impressed new members of the group with the number of battle scars she could talk about from her war with cancer. After some newcomer finished explaining about the developments in their life, and how they viewed having cancer, Artie would often just break in with a curt comment. "Well, I've had four [or five, depending upon the year] different cancers," she would begin. Since her experiences had been so varied she did not talk much about specific adjunctive measures or what to eat. She rarely even thought about exercise. For Artie, the details didn't matter much. This was a battle for survival and principally required a person's commitment. How you chose to fight was of lesser importance, like how you might choose

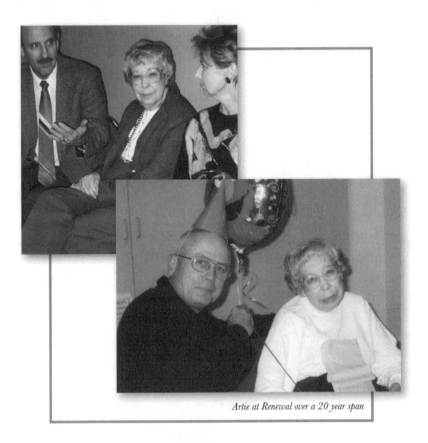

Artie at Renewal over a 20 year span

your own weapon for the fight. Despite this pugnaciousness her comments often contained an element of acceptance about what had happened. She emphasized how she, and by inference, her listener needed to get in touch with reality. Follow the necessary treatment, wherever that takes you, and then focus on getting on with life.

Artie's stated purpose in sharing her experiences with the group was to broadcast encouragement. She wanted you to know that things might seem tough right now, but there is something good awaiting you on the other side of present difficulties. "You're just getting started," came across pretty strong from her to a newcomer. "Do what you have to do. Live as well as you can."

About as deep as Artie ever went in introspection was to talk about living down wind of nuclear tests conducted in the 1940s. Maybe where she lived for several years might have exposed her to nuclear contamination from above-ground detonations. Maybe this was why she had so many troubles to contend with now. "But," she would conclude, "There's nothing to do about that now, is there?"

Artie had been a widow for many years. She had one daughter whom she relied on, especially after the debility accompanying her last treatments. Then the daughter moved to the East Coast for a new job and Artie returned to being self-sufficient and alone. Artie was a great proponent of the municipal senior center. She lived close by and went there every day. The center's schedule became her schedule. It gave added structure to her life. Artie loved to play bridge daily along with whatever activity might be featured at the center. "Well, down at the center…" was a way for her to introduce what had happened in her life during the past week.

After treatment for her fifth cancer Artie was obviously physically impaired. This whole saga had now gone on for almost 20 years. She became visibly stooped and frail. For months she had trouble controlling her saliva, dabbing at the corner of her mouth in a self-conscious way. She now wore more psychological campaign ribbons than anyone in the group. She was our top sergeant based upon her years in the trenches and accepted this seniority in a matter-of-fact way. She made a point of never complaining. Ever. That was just beneath her. She had the little things to talk about to let us know she was still in the fight to maintain her independence. Artie loved coffee. Knowing this, occasionally I would inquire during the long months when she could not swallow. Had she been able to have a cup? "Nope," was the answer for a long time. "I still go down to Starbuck's though," she wanted us to know. "I just go to smell the aroma and keep in practice."

Artie grew weaker over time, partly because she did not eat. She had been our mainstay for years. She finally died peacefully, confident she had risen to contend with everything cancer had thrown at her. And won.

— Trude —

Trude was a woman not unlike Artie. They were about the same age and both exuded a type of confidence when they spoke because of their experience with cancer. The two of them even clashed occasionally in a sort of "Well, I think…Well, I think…" way. Trude usually ended up deferring to Artie in these exchanges because she felt unable to win. She had only two (or three, depending upon how you counted it) different cancers. She lacked the battle ribbons and seniority in experience that Artie had. These were two tough, strong women and Trude still had a lot to say.

Trude had come to the U.S. after marrying an American soldier in Europe following WWII. She was born in Germany in 1928. She met her future husband while he was in the Army overseas. In 1953 they returned to the U.S. and settled in a small town in Washington State. He taught school and she raised their family. In 1980 she was treated with bilateral radical mastectomies for cancer in both breasts. After that she had more surgery to remove additional lymph nodes. This took place prior to the formation of Renewal but she soon found us. Breast cancer was an experience Trude

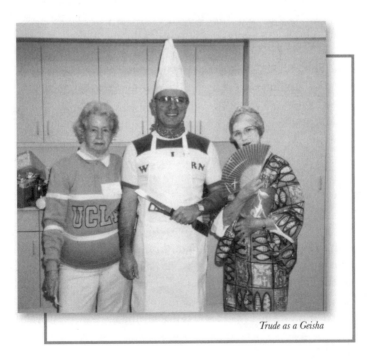

Trude as a Geisha

rarely spoke about. Except for a few self-deprecating references to being flat-chested, she almost never talked about her treatment. In 1987 she was diagnosed with a different cancer, chronic lymphocytic leukemia. This is what prompted her joining our group. She monitored her white blood cell counts as a measure of how she was doing. She was followed closely for any rise in her lymphocyte count. The most common item she had to tell us about was that lab report. Beyond that her interest was in staying well, exploring new ways to do so, and sharing what she learned with Renewal.

One of Trude's memorable contributions to the group was to talk about ways to use scarves when women lose their hair from chemotherapy. This idea is much better known today, but it was something Trude had dreamed up by herself years ago. She carried a collection of colorful pieces of fabric suggesting at the beginning we were about to see some magician's sleight of hand tricks, not a fashion show.

Trude was very animated, fast-talking, and frequently paused to laugh at something she herself had just said. That came across as genuine amusement with self and sort of, "Who knows what I'm going to say next?" Such an approach, plus her varied topics, made for very entertaining contributions. Her enthusiasm spilled over into critiquing subjects discussed at the meetings and the guest speakers.

She wrote lists of subjects important to getting well. She had strong religious beliefs and frequently shared scripture passages and interpretation of things in the Bible. Much of this she either handed off to me at the meetings or mailed to my home. I still have a file of some of her letters. A couple of the thoughts she shared: "People are defeated in life not because of lack of ability, but for the lack of wholeheartedness. They do not wholeheartedly expect to succeed." And: "Let nothing disturb you, let nothing frighten you. Everything passes away except God. God alone is sufficient." In a hand-written note to me in 1986 she wrote, "I hope I don't get on your nerves by being so straight forward! I would like to think I am contributing to the group by being different and enthusiastic."

In another letter she wrote about going to Germany for "fresh cell" injection therapies and to obtain homeopathic drugs from Switzerland. Even so she worried, "But [in so doing] I was a bit like most patients: letting the healing be done to me by someone or something else." She did not condone passivity; she wanted to be calling the shots. Knowing that about Trude makes it easier to understand how enthusiastic she was about the things she could do for herself such as yoga, visualization, and prayer.

Trude was convinced of the efficacy of going to spas and "taking the waters" as a part of therapy. She had an affinity for this more European model of specialized retreats but also found similar facilities to visit in Mexico. About every six months she headed off to some spa in Europe, letting us know before and after what specific benefit she hoped to attain by seeking help on the Continent. As an outgrowth of that travel experience, she gave repeated demonstrations of what to take and how to pack for a month in Europe using one small carry-on bag. It was really an amazing thing. It suggested almost some sleight of hand magic to see how many things went into, and came out of, her little valise. Trude also traveled with a guitar, improbable as that sounds for someone traveling light, but she loved music and loved to play.

Trude's bubbly energy was infectious. She kept us interested in whatever she had to share. She was another of our symbols of independent thinking and determination. She inspired others at the same time she was helping herself. She gradually weakened as the years passed. "She persevered through a lot of negative things," her daughter-in-law recently told me. Trude finally died peacefully, sharing positive advice and optimism until the very end.

— Tom and Jon —

I put these men together to make a point even though these are really two separate stories. Renewal meetings had a lot of openness and sharing, but that was not people sitting around wailing about what fate had dealt them. These two men, like many of the others, were as tough as nails—both physically and mentally. Tom was employed as a hod carrier. He was not an educated man, but had a family and worked hard in supporting them. He spent his work week transporting brick or cement in a wheelbarrow. To hold his hand was like picking up a piece of warm iron. He and others like him were less likely to speak up or to complain at our meetings, but he did attend regularly. Tom had an advanced cancer in his rectum by the time a diagnosis was made. I operated on him. After surgery he had radiation and chemotherapy, but the tumor recurred, as it often does, around the nerves in the pelvis. This is one of the most intractable and painful conditions any cancer patient can face. It is a terribly debilitating trial for someone's courage. Even advanced techniques like implanted nerve stimulators and, finally, cutting pain fibers in the spinal cord failed to relieve Tom's symptoms. He was with us for a long time but ultimately died in our nearby hospice.

Jon had a different personality, more outgoing and jovial, but many of the same physical characteristics as Tom. His profession for over twenty years was operating a jackhammer. All day, every day, he man-handled that heavy piece of equipment, shattering asphalt and concrete in road repair. Jon developed some peculiar loss of feeling in his arms that initially was attributed to his line of work. Physical therapy failed to halt progression of the numbness. Eventually the cause was traced to an obscure tumor right in the central part of his brain stem where it exits from the skull. After much testing and consultation it was the opinion of several experts that surgical removal of Jon's tumor was not technically possible. He was treated with radiation instead.

Jon had a very supportive wife who came to the Renewal meetings with him. She continued working as a waitress even after progressive symptoms forced her husband to retire on disability. She arranged her shift schedule to accompany him. Jon also was not an educated man, but the time he had cancer became the time when his personality began to flourish. He and his wife had one son and the three of them lived in a home in a rural setting. Jon liked to raise exotic evergreen trees, all sorts of bushes and flowers. I got to know him better than some members because of our common interest in plants. Jon was one of the few people of modest means who had been able to create, and live in, a veritable Garden of Eden. His yard was incredible. I bought a truck load of plants from him. He took such an interest in seeing everything done correctly that he came over and helped me place the new plants around my home. I think he was as pleased as I was with the result. After that he often asked if a certain rhododendron had flowered yet, or how another one was growing.

It turned out also that Jon had been interested in playing fiddle for years. After his tumor forced retirement he found a local combo and a spot to fit in and play with them. He started playing gigs with them every weekend at a lively roadhouse bar. That musical talent had to wait a long time to show itself, but for Jon it became a source of real pride and satisfaction. He had realized a dream and become a musician!

Of importance to our story is how Jon participated in the Renewal group discussions. Without any false modesty he was essentially saying, "Look, I'm not an educated man, but this is my life on the line. I have a wife and son and a newfound interest in music. All my doctors say they can't do anything with my case, so now it's up to me."

What he really focused on was doing his own research for things he thought might retard his tumor's growth. Oddly enough the principle thing he settled on was taking shark's cartilage. That was being popularized in some alternative literature at the time. He became our conduit for that information. Jon found a source and took this supplement for many months.

What was the harm? Medical experts had told him they had nothing to offer. In the last years of his life Jon and his wife moved to Oregon where he eventually died. Another of the strong, silent type who didn't conquer his cancer but disease gave him a musical gift and a new perspective on life.

— Priscilla —

Priscilla was a woman with the group mostly remembered for one inspiring story. After her cancer diagnosis and treatment she had a recurrence. This "really had me bummed out" as she would say. As she told the group, she had no idea what to do next. The options presented to her by her physicians were depressing and progressive weakness seemed certain. She shared these concerns in Renewal as her next birthday approached. Her husband inquired about suitable gifts but she responded saying she didn't care. When he insisted she responded with suggestions like maybe a new recliner chair to spend her remaining time more comfortably. Perhaps a tripod cane to help her walk would be good. Maybe he could get her a wheelchair because she probably would need that too.

The next meeting after her birthday Priscilla came to report she was perplexed, even exasperated. The birthday celebration had been over the past weekend. And what had her husband given her? A bicycle! "What am I going to do with a bicycle?" she wondered aloud. But with her husband's encouragement she decided to give cycling a try. It had a wobbly start, but she gradually improved. She reported progressing to riding around the block in her neighborhood. She was weak from treatment, but started to get stronger. She developed more interest in other things she could do to improve her performance, most of them centering on further conditioning for bike riding. Next, Priscilla would report at Renewal, she had gone out and tried a new trail somewhere because it was more interesting than her neighborhood. The story progressed. She started going for more distance. The last report I remember about this new interest in life was when she participated in the Chilly Hilly, a strenuous 33 mile bike ride held each spring on one of the San Juan Islands. She was elated when she was able to complete such a challenge. She spoke of new confidence that sprang from her newly developed sense of fitness.

— Pam H. —

Pam H. is one of so many others who brought a special talent to share with us. She was diagnosed with breast cancer in 1994. While undergoing treatment she developed a melanoma on one arm and that too was excised. As a result of having cancer Pam took up painting. She grew to be a quite accomplished artist and had several shows locally. She helped develop a meditation class at the local hospital and repeatedly taught an advanced version of that class. She showed how to turn the very difficult times of living with cancer into something meaningful. She also developed an "artist's way" class and opened that up to the public. An unusual feature of her work was how she tried to interpret her moods and concepts about cancer on to canvas.

Despite developing a recurrence with bone and liver metastases in 1998 Pam continued to be an active facilitator of Bosom Buddies, the separate women's breast cancer group. She volunteered her services to other community groups including the National Cancer Survivors Day celebrations and often provided special art work for such events. She donated her talents in creating memory books for a support group for kids whose parents had cancer.

What I remember most vividly about viewing her art was how dark, scary even, some of her paintings were. There were jumbled body parts, mouths open in a perpetual cry of anguish. When Pam explained these works to me, though, she was quite upbeat. It was like transferring dark thoughts to canvas got them out of her system, a way of putting them somewhere else. I also remember feeling there was an element of expiation on canvas in what she portrayed, but that never was expressed in words.

What is a bit unusual is how Pam responded to one of my occasional inquiries as to what the group was learning. How was being in Renewal helping move ahead in your life? I really did want to know. It was a self check for me. Pam did not respond immediately. She chose to think this over for some time. Then one day she unexpectedly delivered a hand written letter with the title, "Benefits from support groups." It started with a numbered itemization, but ended with more of a rush of feelings. Her personal account is just that, but it is so clear an expression, instead of writing a biographical sketch as I have done for several others in this chapter, I am having Pam use her own words. She speaks directly to you. So, what is the benefit of a support group?

[Benefit #1 is] Seeing you are not alone in your fear, anxiety, frustration, dread, or in your physical reactions to treatment.

[Benefit #2 is] seeing the range of reactions to cancer and to treatment helps to open your eyes to other possible ways to look at your illness and your treatment.

[Benefit #3 is] seeing other survivors and patients who are in more serious, dire situations than your own. That gives perspective on your own condition. It also allows you to feel relief and gladness that you're in your situation, not theirs. That's a mean thought, perhaps, but natural. You see people in dire circumstances who are coping with it, dealing with it, fighting it, and learning new things from the situation. Perhaps most important, THESE ARE SPUNKY, <u>ALIVE</u> PEOPLE! They are not numb. They are inspiring. I'm grateful to know a person like Artie. What a great attitude! She's had 3 kinds of cancer [which was true at that time in the 1990s] and I've had 2. I'm sure just knowing Artie exists with her 3 cancer diagnoses helped me handle the blow of finding that I had a second type of cancer. Life is fragile and uncertain for every one; we cancer patients/survivors are just more aware of it. And that isn't a bad thing. Anything that increases awareness is a benefit.

Good ideas of new areas to explore come from hearing what other participants have found. Dr. DeShazo's attitude of not condemning any idea as quackery or unlikely to be of benefit helps me. At first so much of alternative treatment seemed dubious to me. Dr. DeShazo told us, any "treatment" might benefit someone, so who is he to say something is worthless? I think it's a combination of belief plus placebo effect. But, hey, if it works for someone, terrific. I came to the Renewal group originally to see how to evaluate more "alternative" ideas that were coming my way. I'd read Bernie Siegel and Lawrence LeShan and O. Carl Simonton and had re-commenced my meditation practice—something I have found to be of immense benefit. But, I didn't know how to judge Essiac tea, vitamins, my diet, CoQ-10, herbs, and things like that.

A man I know called me to say he'd made a device to cure Lyme disease with electromagnetic waves. He wanted me to know he had cured an advanced breast cancer! One case of breast cancer! Well, I've had breast cancer. I've learned to go with what makes sense to me, and what feels right to me. I've learned to trust my intuition about this "medical" area of much importance to my life. I grew up with a Christian Scientist mother. She was totally negative about medicine and doctors—a quite rigid belief system that has not managed her own health problem, Parkinson's disease, well either. I was kept out of classes on science because of her.

In college I visited a doctor for the first time at Planned Parenthood for birth control. I think now that I have given too much trust to allopathic doctors until recently, not realizing how little they know. My doctors in this cancer experience have been terrific, wonderful, caring, and supportive people. I love all three of them. But, I've learned to rely more upon myself to make health decisions. I read lots of medical books about my cancer and about new cancer treatments that are being developed. I now know lots more about how medicine is practiced and about how it is changing. I have a much more independent ability to judge all treatments.

Hindsight being 20-20, I wish I'd never taken hormone replacement therapy for what may have been pre-menopausal insomnia (with no other menopausal symptoms). Maybe I was depressed. Maybe an anti-depressant would have worked. Maybe sleeping pills alternating with anti-histaminics would have been better than estrogen. I don't remember ever hearing about increased incidence of breast cancer with taking estrogen. Of course I was "unlikely" to get breast cancer with no history in my family. I remember hearing about endometrial and ovarian/uterine cancer increase, but there's none of that in my family, either. I wish I'd known more about menopause and hormone replacement therapy. I wish I had known more about HRT and the Pill. And about how little the Pill was really tested. I'm now a much more aware and cautious medical consumer.

I do think that having Dr. DeShazo's medical knowledge present at the meeting helps keep the group grounded and not off on too fantastical stories of miracle cures. The focus is on living well now…learning now.

Many people are afraid of death. I have always been afraid of it. We try to ignore it. Since I came to have cancer I've relaxed a great deal about death. I certainly don't want to die anytime soon. I'd happily live into my 90s and still be making art. That's my goal. But I do see death as yet another experience.

I'm not so terrified anymore. And I don't need to avoid thinking about death. Until then I plan to do a lot of living, doing what I enjoy and what seems meaningful to me. I am a great deal less driven by what other people want of me. I think talking to other people who are facing life-threatening illness and hearing their feelings has contributed to my new attitude.

Pam stayed with her painting. She developed an unusual way of putting art work inside boxes like a diorama. She loved Bruce Springsteen. She took off several times and drove to other states just to dance and celebrate life by attending concerts. She developed an interest in Southwest Native American art and traveled to New Mexico to learn more. She moved to a craftsman-style house in Seattle that she felt was more conducive to her work. At least once she hosted an elaborate Valentine's Day party there for her friends with breast cancer.

Upon learning of her recurrence she developed what she called her "cancer battle plans" and underwent chemotherapy, all the while continuing these varied interests. She died of metastatic disease in 2002.

— Dianne —

Dianne was another woman with a great deal of artistic talent. She sewed and made exquisite dolls and costumes. From time to time there would be an occasion for her to bring in and display her work. She and several others added another dimension to Renewal, for many of us had little or no artistic talent at all. We got to observe close-up how someone could use art for something practical like making money. That was easy to understand. More enlightening was to hear how expressions of art allowed Dianne, and members like her, to convey their concepts of cancer and their journey toward health and normalcy.

— Barbara and Jane O. —

Here is another artificial pairing of two separate people. Both exemplify how life already can be difficult, and then cancer comes along to add to the burden. Jane O. was left by her husband while trying to raise her children. She had essentially no money and no work skills. She was overweight and had troubles with her knees, hips, and back. Life seemed to be just a series of financial problems and dead ends. Her medical course was uneventful but having cancer had introduced a new degree of uncertainty.

I once encountered Jane when I was taking a walk down a lonely country road. We stopped and spent a few minutes chatting before going on our separate ways. Jane actually did not live so very far from that spot and told me, simplistic as it was, she was trying to get some control over her chaotic life and had decided to start with a walking program. I think coming to Renewal helped her quite a bit. It was the one place she could talk in a group of adults instead of just to her kids. People at Renewal actually would be attentive even when she rambled on in an unfocused way. At the time she had no one else in her life to listen. Starting with her walking Jane began to get her life organized. As months passed she spoke more optimistically and began to see some options. The last time she came to a meeting Jane spoke enthusiastically about having just purchased a motorcycle. And now she was going to learn to ride it!

Barbara also had been left by her husband and had no money. She was highly educated, much more articulate and colorful in describing the depth of her despair. She was about 65 when she started coming to Renewal. A recurring theme she expressed was the opinion that life had no future for her. Barbara and her husband had been quite prosperous. Barbara recalled glowing memories of an active social life and travel. Her husband had his own construction business and no money worries. Then, according to Barbara, her husband simply disappeared. Later he resurfaced in Mexico with a much younger woman who had been one of the company's employees. Apparently with some planning the husband had been able to move all his assets out of the country ahead of his departure. By the time the divorce papers arrived there was nothing left to provide for Barbara and her ex-husband was beyond reach. She was reduced to taking a modest apartment and inexpensive car.

So when Barbara spoke to Renewal it was principally about the difficulty she had in contending with her new life without money. There was never enough money. She could no longer do any of the things she used to enjoy. Giving up vacations and every other sort of travel was a big issue. The fact that she had been treated for breast cancer, and having to face that alone, was sort of like the last straw. Compared to the indignity of her situation cancer was relegated to being an incidental detail but of course she worried about it. More immediate was worry about her face, neck, and her hands. Barbara had sun damage sustained in decades of trips to exotic places during her marriage. Now she had recurring troubles with both squamous and basal cell cancers. Multiple excisions caused scars that left her feeling disfigured and worrying about what was coming next.

Once again I credit the general course of Renewal meetings with helping this lady. Barbara still had much to say about "that son of a bitch who left me penniless," but she also began to join in the more positive themes of self help. She began to accept what had happened with her marriage. She moved on to a more positive interest in what was happening now. There were several other socially prominent women at our meetings. Barbara came to see that they might not have her same financial worries, but some had physical afflictions and disfigurement far worse than her own.

When we started looking for a place to have demonstrations of healthy cooking it was Barbara who volunteered first. Each time we went to Barbara's apartment she offered excuses for her modest, subsidized living quarters. The group responded with only compliments for her comfortable home. She began to see her living space in a new light and finally stopped making apologies.

One week Barbara proudly announced she was making a trip to the East Coast to visit relatives. The members understood what breakthrough thinking this represented and congratulated her. The next year we heard a similar announcement about an upcoming trip to Europe. The trips Trude was making to Europe despite a very limited budget seemed to be part of the impetus for Barbara. This improvement in Barbara's financial picture was never explained. I suspect it was more perception than monetary in nature. Over several years the victim role and the bitterness subsided. Barbara accepted the skin cancer problem in a new, matter-of-fact way. She continued on with the group in a more contented way until she died suddenly of a heart attack on one of her new traveling adventures.

— Four Women Who Did Too Much —

If I am to be totally honest in this book, I have to confess that I was not all-knowing in leading Renewal. And there were things I missed hearing about and other things I did not understand. For now let this admission be personified by four women in the group:

The first of these was one of the initial people outside my practice to join the original Renewal group. She was a registered nurse, relatively young, smart, and quite organized in her thinking. Organized I was not, so when this woman I didn't know offered to become our group secretary I thought it was a great idea. She had been treated for breast cancer in another city and never volunteered much about her clinical history. In the months after we started meeting she did a great job. She got the membership organized. She took names and addresses, organized a phone tree, arranged refreshments. She personally called people when they missed a meeting to find out if they were OK. She would then call and let me know the latest update if she felt the news shouldn't wait until the next meeting. She really helped us get off to a good start and everyone came to rely upon her. By the end of her first year with the group she began to look bad. Her face was tired and drawn and she lost weight. She, our first secretary, died in less than a year. She was doing so much for me and the group I always felt afterwards I should have been more attuned to her needs in assessing what was obviously a recurrence of her cancer.

— Pat —

A second woman took over as secretary after that. This woman, Pat, was much more easy-going and had a wonderful manner of talking to people as individuals. She let each person know she cared about them. It was a nice complement to the open discussions to have Pat make mental notes about things for follow-up. She had a good sense about when to offer help to an individual with some problem and when to leave them alone. She also had been treated for breast cancer elsewhere with a lumpectomy and radiation. I wouldn't have known much about her clinical history if she hadn't come to see me once for a second opinion. Her follow-up with her physician had suggested a local recurrence within the breast.

Pat wanted to know what I thought. Her surgeon had now recommended a mastectomy for the recurrence. After my examination and reviewing all the tests I concurred. I told her that was the best idea. It was evident that this middle-aged woman considered her breasts her best physical asset. She did in fact have ample, attractively contoured breasts and I knew having the left one removed would be hard. She said in our discussion that she'd have to think about my advice. My intuition told me this was her way of saying, No.

What I didn't appreciate at the time was that Pat felt ambivalent because she knew her husband enjoyed her physical appearance. Later I found out Pat had confided to another woman in the group that she felt giving up something her husband enjoyed so much would not be fair to him. How much difference her decision made, of course, I don't know. I do know that Pat kept on being our unofficial secretary for quite some time and was as industrious as ever. My cautions to her about not overdoing were non-specific and never seemed to lead to any change. When her recurrent disease finally did overtake her, she stayed with us, sharing actively what was happening until close to the time she died. I remember the months she carried on, acting unchanged, but seeming sad as if she knew she'd soon be gone.

— Martha —

Martha is the third of the women mentioned. She too was with the group for years. She was always quiet, almost apologetic about getting cancer. She hinted she felt this wasn't just her disease; it inconvenienced everyone who knew her. She always said she was alone but in fact had two sisters. This was only part of the complexity of relationships I did not know. Afterwards I wondered if I had spent more time with her, might I have changed the course of events.

The thing most people remember about Martha is her dog. She was a very giving person and had gone through quite a process to have her dog, a golden retriever, trained to be a comfort dog for people who are ill. Training isn't really the right word. It's at least partly recognizing a sort of empathy in a dog (or cat) just like seeing empathy demonstrated in people. Dogs like hers intuitively know how to come into a room with a sick or dying person and comfort them just by staying nearby. I wish more people could understand how meaningful that can be. Many such animals know instinctively when someone is about to die. If a dog like Martha's is taken on a hospice ward it will choose what you'd say is the most appropriate patient room on its own. You can be sure that the person in that room will be the next one to die.

Martha and her dog became a resource for the hospice staff to call upon. She also brought her dog to some Renewal meetings. It would lie near her chair and watch attentively as people spoke. Sometimes the dog would get up and go over to someone and nuzzle like she wanted to be petted. But it wasn't a needy thing; it was more like the dog detected who was having a difficult moment and knew what to do. We weren't dealing with imminent death at Renewal, but the members always responded warmly to Martha's dog.

Martha was closer to her dog than to any human, I suppose. That was something I did not appreciate. Nor was I privy to the extent of Martha's cancer recurrence. She was too private a person to let a whole group like ours come into her world.

Then the dog was killed in an accident. About that time it became known that Martha was dealing with a recurrence.

Martha did have a network of women friends I had never met. Martha let her friends know she was unwilling to continue on a slow downhill course. She decided upon assisted suicide and then she and these friends all moved along together in a knowing way. Most of Renewal and I only found out about these details at the touching memorial her friends and sisters gave. I felt a sense of loss that suicide was not avoided but most people concluded it was clearly the way Martha wanted to go.

Martha chose to be cremated. At her memorial there were two urns of ashes on the altar, hers and her dog's.

The final of these four is not someone we knew well in the group, but in the theme of what I am trying to convey here, she deserves mention. This woman in her late 60s just appeared at Renewal as people sometimes did. She told everyone she had been a smoker and drinker in the past. She never supplied details, but had been treated with surgery for lung cancer. As I listened to her in the passing weeks I put her in my category of Wise Women. Here was someone who had been through much and learned a great deal from her experiences. She was substantiation of how valuable past or present alcoholics can be once they find a way to compensate.

This woman came to the fore one time when we were discussing our phone tree. People liked the fact they knew there were others in the group they could call on if they had a need. Some formed associations and friendships just to chat outside the structure of our regular meetings. It was on this point this older woman weighed in. She told us how she made it a habit to stay in phone contact with a broad network of all sorts of people. Because of her lung damage she rarely went out. Coming to our meetings was a chore, but she did have a suggestion to make: it was her lifestyle to be awake most of the night, especially late at night. I think this was because she couldn't breathe well lying down. And I suspected from her husky voice and actions that she still smoked heavily and stayed awake much of the time just to have another cigarette. She was on the other side of the learning curve about the association of smoking with health problems. She was going down and didn't think much about it.

Her suggestion was this: If we went forward with some sort of resource list of people willing to take calls, why not let her take the night shift? "Since I'm awake every night anyway, why don't you let me take calls from midnight to say, six a.m.?" She was sincere, but I weighed in that I didn't think that was a good idea. I told her she needed to focus more on taking care of her self and devote the night to getting rest.

That made sense to me the physician, but not to her, the Renewal member. I probably was projecting too much of the role of patient upon her. I think that was the last Renewal meeting she attended. We, or I, wouldn't honor what she thought she uniquely had to offer so she moved on. She went back to her apartment in Seattle and the network of her other contacts. We phoned her a few times, but she died not long after.

I came to realize I looked upon losing a Renewal member much the same way I looked upon losing one of my surgical patients. The time to die comes to everyone, but I still didn't like it. I struggle to accept that I personalized this too much. For these four women just mentioned I feel they were looking more for meaning and being useful rather than for help with disease. I hoped for some opportunity for them to reach acceptance. Still, what was being lost was not something that was mine to lose.

Describing these four women as a composite brings them to your attention and mine. It is a reminder to be vigilant in group work. Situations are not always what they seem. What I learned here was that as each of us approaches our own specific illness we must become intimate with the pain in our heart. We should not try to get away from it.

We think we can attend to the pain and troubles of others and distance ourselves from our own pain, but we cannot. This is true despite the fact that avoiding personal pain is the very model of health care we have created in this country. A person avoiding their own pain will not be successful as they hope to be. Such a person may become angrier trying to avoid discovering the source of his or her pain than from dealing with disease diagnosis. Such futile effort consumes energy. It leads to exhaustion and burnout. And, it postpones our renewal.

— Pam R. —

As we conclude this chapter I won't say that I have saved the best until last. Every person remembered here has value just like their stories do. Still, I will say that the story that Pam related about herself was one of the most memorable in Renewal. It came about in the early years of our meetings yet is still one of the first that comes to my mind. Other members remember Pam also as "that woman who had the brain tumor" even when they have forgotten her name. And, this story continues even up to the present time.

There are at least three things that come to mind when I remember Pam. First, her presence. She just started appearing at our meetings and relating her story. She had the appearance of an average woman and lived in a nearby town in one sense, but she had a conviction, an overriding certainty about who she was, that could not be missed. Second, she had a certainty about what she had done. She left an indelible impression upon people hungry for success stories and gave them hope. Some readers will find such a conclusion unsupported and scoff. I hope you will not be so cynical as to reject the hope. Third, I took note that Pam came to us after the fact. By the time we saw her, what she accomplished was already an established fact. In the usual sense Renewal did not help her. She helped us. She came to see us just as Saga One was ending. She was just finding her voice to talk to others.

Pam is part of what, early on, convinced me one day I would be writing this book.

Finding Pam wasn't easy. She did not stay in Renewal long and it had been almost 25 years since I had seen her. She had moved several times, leaving only a trace memory here and there. I began to think she was dead. It took help from several people for me to finally track her down. Even though she had moved and been away for years, she had returned to live in Seattle. When I called her in 2008 we had this wonderful talk where she reaffirmed everything I remembered. Then she added quite a bit more.

Pam was diagnosed with a brain tumor in 1983. She had increasing trouble with headaches and neck aches. Then she started having seizures as frequently as three to five times a day. She also had trouble remembering everyday things. Pam went to the University Hospital with her complaints. X-rays were done, and then an angiogram confirmed the extent of involvement. She was told it was a tumor, and very large.

"How large?" she asked.

"Why do you want to know?" one of the doctors questioned her back.

"It's important for me to know," she insisted.

So they told her in layman's terms, "It's the size of a small grapefruit." That was their approximation. They told her this was too large to be removed surgically. Later an open brain biopsy did confirm that this was an astrocytoma, a type of malignancy. After a quarter century, Pam doesn't remember any more about the clinical aspects of the tumor than that.

What Pam was thinking at the university she didn't say. About a year later at Renewal she was telling us as part of her story. She needed to know how big this thing was if she was going to defeat it. She had to be able to see it with her mind's eye. The brain biopsy was done just before Christmas. After that she started on a course of radiation therapy to her brain.

What Pam said then and told me again now was essentially, the doctors did what they were going to do and I did what I was going to do. "Once I could see this grapefruit in my head, I could see it was made up of thousands of little particles, like sand. So all I had to do was start dissolving those little particles and the tumor would get smaller." The exact rate, and the objective oversight with CT scans is a bit hazy, but the essential story is what she told us at Renewal: "So gradually, the tumor began to shrink. First it got to the size of an orange. Then it was a tennis ball, then it became a golf ball, then finally it was the size of a marble."

This was an unexpected development, even though the physicians had done what they intended and hit the growth with radiation. "They couldn't explain this," Pam remembers. "Then, when they told me it was as small as a marble, I kept on taking away these grains of sand. It kept getting smaller and smaller. "Remember that statement in the bible about faith as big as a grain of mustard seed? Well, I saw this thing going down to that size." Then, one day, she continued, "I knew it was gone." She went in for her next appointment and announced that the tumor was gone. Another CT scan confirmed there was no tumor visible. "None of my doctors could believe it."

Some time after these revelations Pam stopped coming to Renewal. Many of us still remember because this was our most graphic story of success with visualization up until that time. Pam had always seen herself as a positive person and that is what she feels made her visualization succeed.

Move forward 25 years and Pam is telling this same story to me again. She added some personal facts: She had married the first time at age 18 and had three children, then divorced. When she had this experience with the brain tumor she was 38 years old. After the events of 1983 she married a second time and had a fourth child. One son has died.

She also made an addition to her story, grounded in that time in 1983, but she did not talk about it then. She only has come to talk about it now because what happened has occured twice. "I've been up to heaven twice," she tells me calmly. "One day as I was coming out from an appointment at University Hospital [in 1983] my husband was driving and he stopped to pick me up. All of a sudden I was just lifted up. I went somewhere. And then a voice said, 'You are very sick, but don't worry. You'll come back from this…take care.' And that was it," she concludes, "I knew from that moment that I could make the tumor disappear, and I did."

Pam bridged across to what came later by saying, "After that I felt very confident about visualization. I knew I could make bad things go away whenever anything happened. Just make it a bunch of mustard seeds."

In 1994 she started having trouble again. She returned to the University Medical Center. "I had the best doctor," she brightens up as we talk. "He said I had another brain tumor, on the other side. This one was on the left side, in the area of the motor cortex and speech. It was big but he thought we should try to remove it. [Giving radiation treatment twice is not considered safe.] This was an odd one, an oligodendroma. He told me he removed a quarter of my brain."

Pam had been warned that after the operation she would not be able to use the right side of her body or speak. "They told me I would be in a wheel chair from then on." Pam gave me an aside, "My dad had been in a wheel chair for 25 years. There was no way I was going to be in a wheel chair the rest of my life!" So she got up after surgery very quickly. "On the third day I got out of that wheel chair and took a cane. I never went back." She does not dismiss the need for rehabilitation. "I had to relearn how to walk. My right arm didn't work so I had to exercise that too. And, I got my speech back." Some troubles linger on after 14 years: "I still can't read very well." Then she adds optimistically, "But I keep practicing; I'm reading more all the time."

Now about that second trip to heaven: "I'm no kook," she warned me. "But I got taken up to heaven again. It was after I got back home from the second surgery. I got up one night to go to the bathroom. I heard a voice and thought it was my husband calling to me. So I tried to turn on the light." Pam is purposefully vague about this, but what she said was, "Then I realized there were two angels, one on each side, and they lifted me up. They took me up and it was like I was in the clouds. They brought me up to see my Maker, and a voice said, 'My child, my child, you are back here for a reason.' Then He said, "This time you are cured. This time you have to tell the world. You have a mission. Speak from your heart." Then she was back. She got into bed again but felt like she had been struck by lightning.

Pam abruptly changed the subject and asked me, "How many people have you talked to that have lost a quarter of their brain?" She didn't have to wait for my answer and continued, "Now I talk to people, I give them love and hope. I tell them to give love back to others. Giving love is why we are here."

"I have changed so much," Pam continued, "I do my yoga every day. I have changed my diet a lot to eat grains and nutritional foods. I know I sound like an old foggie—but I'm talking about eating the way we did when we were children at home." Pam is 63 now. There are still challenges. "My second husband decided he didn't want to be married any more and left me. I have balancing exercises to do every day because my balance still is not good." She fell six months ago and is still dealing with the consequences of that. It's been slow.

"I feel great," she said. "You'd never know I had two cancers. People look at my face and don't believe me. I spend my time giving speeches and writing about my experiences." She had to give up the talks after she fell, but the writing continues. Her website is www.DawningOfMyNewLife. com.

"I'm doing a book about what happened to me. Until I think of something better, I call it *I'd Rather be Better than Bitter.*" Yes, indeed.

CHAPTER 3

FAMILY STORIES

"I went to Renewal with my father and sat next to an older man who could have been my grandfather. When my father introduced himself to the group and started talking about his cancer, I started to cry. The older man put his arm around me and whispered, 'Don't cry now that he's alive. Enjoy him, laugh, have fun with him…cry later.'"
— *Clara B.,*
a young physician who visited Renewal

In this chapter several stories emphasize the support given to a Renewal member by a person close to them. Some of the people in the previous chapter had a spouse or other relative, but their struggle came across more as a solitary effort. That's why they are in Chapter 2. Stories related here demonstrate how important it can be to have someone to relate to and depend upon every day, not just people you see once a week at Renewal. Good relationships cause good things to happen even when contending with cancer.

"Wear me as a seal upon your heart…
for love is strong as death…
Many waters cannot quench love,
no flood can sweep it away…"
— Song of Songs 8:6-7
The New English Bible

— Nancy and Bill —

Bill wrote their story about Renewal for inclusion in this book. Nancy died a number of years ago and Bill has since remarried.

I met Nancy during our junior year in high school. She was a cheerleader and I was co-captain of the football team. I was attracted to her from many perspectives but mostly to her bubbly personality and physical attributes. She was quite an athlete and in great shape physically. She had to be good in order to become a cheerleader in a school with a very successful athletics program. We began dating while in high school. Our growing friendship morphed into a courtship that continued on after graduation, becoming an on-and-off affair for several years. All this finally culminated with our getting married in southern California. We were far away from our families and friends in Connecticut where we came from. Our two children, Marcus and Dena, were born soon after we settled down.

Nancy was always quite active. She was thin, healthy, had lots of energy, and was always involved in something, especially things with our children. In their school she constantly volunteered as a teacher's aid, with Dena's ballet classes and performances, and with Marcus' ice hockey team. She was his team's manager for several years, including making their travel arrangements and all other team functions. Nancy was also very busy with friends, many of whom we considered part of our new, extended, growing family. This latter aspect of our life was critical in that we both came from large, cohesive families. The fact that they all lived on the East coast was always a challenge and one that would became more difficult as the children got older. When the kids got into their own activities and friendships, travel to visit family became less frequent. The friendships developed where we lived would prove to be invaluable. I might add that throughout this period all of our family enjoyed excellent health.

After spending 12 years in California we made a major decision and, subsequently, a humungous move to Issaquah, Washington in 1980. Issaquah was a small town in the suburbs of Seattle. While on a mini vacation there, and on a whim, we purchased a brand new home in a new development and that became our new home. It was literally in the middle of the woods. When we considered what life in California had become for our family, especially in terms of the smog and congestion, the beauty of the Pacific Northwest, with gorgeous mountains and greenery, was pretty compelling. After the trauma of the relocation, we jumped into all the Northwest had to offer. We loved the outdoors and as a family spent as much time as possible exploring the hidden nooks and crannies all over the Northwest. We had our own camping trailer and jeep. We also made good use of the unlimited selection of great hiking trails and picnicking spots throughout the area, especially in the Cascade Mountains.

Marcus took to fly fishing on our trips to Montana. He also was excited to continue with his ice hockey career. It was a wonderful gift for us as well as a real challenge. As his skating skills improved, so did his desire to get more involved in the sport. He quickly advanced to the traveling team where every other weekend we traveled to a rink north of the border for quality competition. The travel to Canada got old but exploring Vancouver and Vancouver Island was a real joy. This travel combined with early morning ice hockey practices kept all of the family quite busy. This was especially true for Nancy. She loved getting involved with the social aspects of the kids' extracurricular activities. Life was busy, active, fun.

We had every reason to believe the upcoming 1986 would be a good year. Marcus' hockey career and Dena's ballet had voluntarily come to an end. Both kids were now getting more involved in school activities and with friends. Everything seemed normal except that Nancy began to complain of discomfort in her right lower abdomen. She experienced this for some time before mentioning it. She didn't want to make a big deal about it or alarm the rest of us.

Nancy's primary medical practitioner was her gynecologist. She brought this discomfort to his attention when she was in for her annual physical examination. She saw him several more times. The sensation, the discomfort, was difficult to describe. The pain persisted, but the doctor could not seem to identify the cause even after extensive testing at his clinic. The doctor finally ordered an ultrasound of Nancy's gallbladder. That seemed to be the closest to the area she felt the discomfort. The test results showed there were some granules in her gallbladder that could be the cause. The doctor recommended she have her gallbladder removed and Nancy agreed.

The surgery was routine. Nancy had no complications although her recovery was slow. This was the first time since her pregnancies that Nancy had been laid up for any length of time, and she didn't like it. After a few months she was feeling better and mostly healed from the surgery. Still the original discomfort that led to the surgery was there. It was in the same area of the abdomen, just below the rib cage on the right. Nancy was getting frustrated. Later we looked back at this time as the beginning of subtle signs that she was slowing down. She had less energy and paid more attention to this continued discomfort. This had an effect psychologically. It was hard for Nancy not to focus on what was going on with her physically. We had all assumed that removing her gallbladder would have eventually solved all her problems.

In September of 1986, with no improvement in her symptoms, we decided Nancy needed to see another doctor, perhaps a specialist. We arranged to see a gastroenterologist who happened to be my primary care doctor. This new consultant did a number of tests of the stomach, esophagus, lower GI tract, and additional blood tests. Again nothing was found that would account for the discomfort as Nancy described it. The doctor finally ordered an x-ray of her lungs and upper GI tract.

Nancy's mom was visiting with us over the Labor Day weekend. Her mother accompanied Nancy to the doctor's office and then to the hospital to have these last tests. The two of them remained at the hospital for the report. The doctor came to the hospital and told both Nancy and her mother about the tests. After that was over the two of them drove home. When they arrived back at the house it was late in the afternoon. I noticed that both of them were subdued and concerned. Nancy said the doctor told her the x-ray showed there was a mass in her left lung. He told her it could be mucous caused by a virus but perhaps something else. Because it was unclear, he scheduled a needle biopsy to get a determination as to what the mass was.

Nancy was upset. The rest of us felt numb. It was hard for Nancy to look at me. I knew if she did she would fall apart emotionally. Her mom was also unable to stay focused. What I heard was frightening—no, shocking. I needed to know more, but didn't know how to ask questions. We all knew this was not good but were too overcome with uncertainty to do anything but remain silent.

The next week after an anxious Labor Day weekend I accompanied Nancy to the hospital where the needle biopsy was scheduled to be done. She wasn't very talkative that morning, just tried to keep busy doing things until it was time to go. While we were at the hospital she spent a lot of that time staring off into space. She had no expression on her face but obviously was in deep thought. To complicate things, the procedure did not go well. There was a partial collapse of her lung while they were trying to obtain samples, not only from the mass in her left lung, but also from what now appeared to be tumors in the right lung.

While Nancy remained in the procedure room after completion of the biopsy, several doctors and technicians gathered around the x-ray view box looking at the pictures. I was close enough to see them. They all had looks of seriousness, almost disbelief, as they discussed what they were seeing. After a time one of the doctors beckoned me over for a look. He told me Nancy was in trouble. The doctors were very sympathetic, but stated in very real terms that Nancy was facing an impossible dilemma. They were also genuinely amazed that someone with the condition they were seeing could look so good physically. She still looked like a normal healthy person.

The x-ray revealed a completely different story. Her left lung was almost white, filled with a mass. There were several tumors in the right lung of various sizes, some also quite large. The doctors were certain Nancy was facing a lung cancer diagnosis. They also detected spots on her spine. They said these were the likely cause of the discomfort she complained about for so long. They said it was something known as referred pain: the cancer in her spine was causing nerve pain to be felt where she noticed it in her abdomen.

After the procedure Nancy was taken to a recovery room to await results of the pathology report and consultation with our doctor. Once again everything was silent. Nancy was uncomfortable but didn't want to talk and I was still numb. I felt unable to focus and found it hard to say anything. I was in shock at what I saw and what the doctors said. What would the future likely be for Nancy, me, and the children? That went through my mind but I couldn't let Nancy see me upset. It was better for me not to get into a conversation.

When the doctor finally came into the room, he appeared solemn. He also looked a bit frazzled and uncomfortable himself. He immediately began to describe to Nancy what had occurred with the biopsy, the problem with the lung collapsing, and what that meant. Then he went right into telling her that the pathology report confirmed what they feared. She had cancer in both lungs. The big mass was in the left lung with seven tumors in the right. There also were three metastases to the spine. He told Nancy he was sorry but that the cancer was inoperable and her condition terminal.

In the shock of this news, Nancy was actually calm. She acted almost prepared. She asked the doctor how much time she had and what she could do. His reply was pretty straight forward; he told Nancy she shouldn't expect to live more than 6 months, perhaps less. He told her she should get her affairs in order. I remember his comment hit right in the core of her being. Nancy was 44. She was petrified, but she was angry too. That caused her to spark back at him and say, "So what am I supposed to do, go home and die?"

The 30 mile ride home was mostly in silence. We still felt numb. We also were in shock and disbelief—everything all at the same time. How do you put something like this into meaningful context? Just a few days ago this young family had a future and it was bright and seemingly predictable. Suddenly, everything turned to bleakness and dread. The impact of this news was profound on both of us. But it wasn't long before Nancy began to react with anger at what she had just heard. It all came rolling out as we drove home, "I don't feel like I'm dying...I still have a lot of living to do...I'm too young to die...What about the kids...Why?"

Thankfully, when we arrived home from the hospital, Nancy's mom was waiting for us, prepared to accept some awful news. She had an inkling of what was going on. Nancy told her mother the diagnosis and prognosis. Her mom tried her best to be reassuring but it was obviously hard for her to contemplate the loss of her daughter. In the days that followed her mother was a blessing to us all, especially to Nancy. At that moment Nancy needed her mother's love and understanding. Later, when the children were home and we were all together, we told them what we knew. The children were 16 and 14 and I've never been sure of their capacity to absorb and fully understand the reality of what they heard, but they tried to be reassuring to their mother. I believe they understood and didn't want to add to Nancy's grief.

On a subsequent follow-up visit with the doctor a week later, we heard about the tumor board at the hospital. We heard the tumor board reviews difficult cases like Nancy's with the goal of determining reasonable treatment options. Our doctor said this board had met and unfortunately confirmed what we had already been told. The board concluded that there were no surgery or treatment options available for such an advanced case of cancer.

Nancy heard this loud and clear. She emphatically heard the "terminal" in the prognosis. When he finished talking Nancy asked anyway if the doctor would recommend an oncologist or radiologist for her to see. She just wanted to talk with someone herself to see if they could help. Our doctor suggested we call an oncologist who happened to be on the tumor board that week when Nancy's case was reviewed. He would already be familiar with her situation. We made the appointment and soon met this wonderful doctor. He seemed genuinely interested in Nancy's dilemma.

Despite the severity of her disease he felt it was possible that chemotherapy could help to reduce or stall the tumor growth. This was great news for all of us but especially for Nancy. She needed to see a little light, a ray of hope. A schedule was established for her to begin receiving chemo treatments. This process, with some changes in the drug protocol along the way, would continue for a long time.

The first treatment, an IV drip in the office, went well. We waited to see how well she would tolerate the chemicals, whether she would experience side effects and of course, whether the treatment had any effect. Unfortunately, Nancy's body did not like the chemicals. Vomiting came the day after infusion and persisted for a couple of days following each treatment. When the vomiting subsided she remained exhausted almost until the next treatment began. This didn't help her appetite or weight but she was so determined to take the treatments and hopeful that they would be effective, she persisted in spite of the side effects.

The first evaluation visit with the oncologist a few weeks later showed some tumor shrinkage. We were all ecstatic. Yes, it was a hard journey, but Nancy saw promise. She was determined to see it through. At every visit, the oncologist ended leaving Nancy with hope. He continued to do this even after there was no tumor shrinkage and even some noticeable tumor growth.

It was during the early part of her illness that Nancy began to show signs of developing anxiety. It was subtle at first, but became more and more of a problem for her and for the rest of the family. Maybe it began as a consequence of the negative reaction she had to the chemotherapy. That was when the vomiting was so bad and Nancy became afraid to drive. She was afraid she might become ill and have to vomit while behind the wheel. This anxiety grew to such a point she would not drive across any of the many bridges in the Seattle area. Eventually she quit driving into Seattle at all. Nancy became increasingly nervous, almost to the point of paranoia, about leaving our house or being in the company of people other than family. Planning any outing, especially if it involved driving somewhere, became tedious. Nancy required a great deal of time and meticulous planning before setting out to go anywhere.

This all began during a special time for both Marcus and Dena. They were preparing to obtain driving permits and began taking driver's education at school. Even many years later the two of them remember this with

mixed emotion. They still recall some of the episodes with their mom trying to help teach them to drive the rural roads of our neighborhood. At
first neither of the children had any understanding of what to do when
behind the wheel. Each of the teenagers had their own anxiety about this.
What they felt was compounded by Nancy's apprehension about every
moment and the oppressive atmosphere it created. In one such outing with
his mom Marcus became so frustrated he slammed on the car brakes, got
out, and walked home.

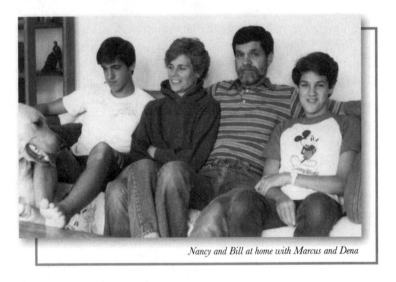

Nancy and Bill at home with Marcus and Dena

It was during this time that we became aware of the Renewal Group
at a local hospital. Someone told us it was a support group for cancer
patients, and Nancy decided to attend a meeting. The group already had
been in existence for several years, and had a reputation for providing good
information to those in the battle. The doctor who organized the group
in the early 1980s welcomed Nancy to the group. Other group members
greeted Nancy with openness and warmth. Nancy was immediately attracted to the camaraderie she witnessed. The group was a collage of colorful individuals. They were from every walk of life and facing myriad
serious physical problems.

Everyone came to the meetings week after week with the same objective: to beat a disease that was busy at work every day attempting to take
their lives. The group was bringing cancer patients together to support each
other by encouraging them to share their life stories, their disease and their

treatment modalities. They talked about their diets, nutrition in general, medications, vitamin supplementation, and any other information they could share. They had lively discussions about anything that could possibly be helpful. It struck me as a mutual quest to get healthy. The group also brought in special guests, doctors and other professionals, with expertise in a particular area to help educate the group on issues of nutrition, alternative medicine, or exercise. It was fortunate that during this time I was able to accompany Nancy to her doctor appointments, for treatments, and to Renewal. I often left Renewal meetings filled with useful information myself. For me it was great fodder. What I learned often times led to more exploratory research on the computer at home or at the library.

Nancy was to build incredibly deep relationships with many at Renewal. This was a special group of people all bonded by a life-threatening dilemma. She found additional inspiration and strength here to continue on. She herself became an inspiration as she never lost her bubbly personality and her energy to help someone when she could. She spent untold hours on the phone helping and being helped by other members of the group.

It was at Renewal we were introduced to macrobiotics. It is a Japanese dietary regimen and way of living that seemed to make a lot of sense to both Nancy and me. With the information picked up at Renewal, I began to spend a lot of time researching macrobiotics at the library and on the internet. Later I bought several books by noted experts Michio Kushi and George Ohsawa, including some with recipes. After trying out some dishes and purchasing some esoteric ingredients, we eventually adopted this regimen as our more or less regular way of eating. We also tried living simply. Looking back, I admit it was mostly my initiative. The dietary transition was not an easy one for the family to make. It was basically a vegetarian regimen that allowed fish, but no dairy or refined sugars. It focused primarily on various robust grains, seeds and nuts, as its basis. Fresh vegetables are prepared in various ways and some fruits are allowed.

Nancy had been a consumer of large quantities of dairy for years so this change seemed like a good one to try. My research indicated that excessive dairy and refined sugars could cause the immune system to weaken, not a good thing for a cancer patient. As I enjoyed cooking and we regularly grew a vegetable and herb garden, it was easy for me to become engrossed in learning more about this regimen. I cooked our meals with lots of fresh produce and using new things like brown rice and sea vegetables. I believe this diet made a dramatic change for all of us. Like a lot of families with children we all consumed our share of ice cream and products loaded with refined sugar. My substitution of other sweeteners in cooking and baking with brown rice syrup and barley malt wasn't always appreciated, however, especially in the cookies. Nancy and the children still preferred ice cream to Rice Dream. I was proud of what came out of the kitchen in spite of the comments from Nancy and the children. They often referred to my cookies as hockey pucks and rapped them on the table to show how hard they were.

We brought cookies to Renewal to share. Nancy had fun mocking them with her peers in the group. Still they all enjoyed eating them and asked me to bring more. Marcus later would recall the times his mother would encourage him, prod him, to request a family trip to McDonalds. Nancy wanted to enjoy an order of fries and have a break from brown rice. I really wanted to participate in Nancy's battle in every way I could. There's no question she also endured the dietary regimen to placate her husband.

Along the same lines Renewal was introduced to something called Biogenics, a most interesting way of living. The presentation at a Renewal meeting taught us the benefits of adding sprouts to the diet, for the powerful boost they provide to maintaining a functional immune system. Nancy was interested in this too. So we became alfalfa sprout farmers and our kitchen an alfalfa sprout farm. We put sprouts on just about everything, from salads to sandwiches. Since Nancy was dealing with lung cancer we also learned about the benefits of vitamin A and beta carotene. She became a big fan of carrots and carrot juice. Before long we were juicing daily and 25 pound bags of fresh carrots didn't last us long. At times Nancy was consuming such a large quantity of carrots it affected her skin color, giving it an orange tone.

Throughout all of this Nancy demonstrated time and again a powerful determination. She wanted to be a cancer survivor. She never stopped being the consummate mom, just added survival skills to life's routine tasks. All the while we were making a lot of dietary and supplement changes learned at Renewal. Nancy continued to receive chemotherapy treatments. Then it became necessary to add radiation treatments to the spine to reduce the tumors there and the pain they caused. It seemed to make it easier for Nancy to have this group she could report to each week, even when the news was not good.

We all knew Dr. DeShazo had started Renewal based upon the influence of Dr. Bernie Siegel, a surgeon in New Haven, CT, who had started a similar group. Dr. Siegel had written about that group's experience and his philosophy in *Love, Medicine & Miracles.* The book was mentioned regularly at Renewal and was one of the books in the lending library. From what she heard, Nancy became interested, especially regarding references to the power of the mind and the use of focused meditation and visualization as a tool in fighting tumor. She got a copy of the book and became engrossed in Dr. Siegel's writing. The book had many stories of individuals like Nancy and the others at Renewal. Those stories proved to be a tremendous support for Nancy. Renewal's library also introduced many other authors. Nancy became interested and pursued material published by several of them including Carl and Stephanie Simonton, and their book *Getting Well Again.* As a result of what she learned from these authors, Nancy established a relationship with a psychologist who had developed and used relaxation tapes as part of his therapy. These tapes became a great comfort to her when she needed to escape from the discomfort of the chemotherapy or the pain from the spinal involvement.

Nancy spent a lot of time with Dr. Siegel's book and his other messages, such as getting on the path to achieving peace of mind. On a scheduled trip to Connecticut, I brought her copy of his book with me. I left it at Dr. Siegel's office in New Haven as instructed by his staff. Knowing the trip was coming I had called his office, explained Nancy's dilemma, and asked if Dr. Siegel would be willing to autograph her book as a surprise for her. He wrote a short note in the book and sent it back to us.

Dr. Siegel also encouraged Nancy to do drawings, a big part of his philosophy for cancer patients. He used the knowledge gained by drawing to help equip patients to fight the disease. He explained utilizing powers within themselves, including visualization. Nancy sent several of her drawings to Dr. Siegel in early 1987. He responded with thoughtful analytical insight for her to consider. About the drawings he wrote back about the first one, "You look little and lost in the doctor's office—solid little person but alone, without contacts or personal relationship. Treatment is good and doctor has a lot to offer, but more than is in his books and diploma. Let treatment in; it is good for you and will change you in a positive direction. Where is your immune system and white cells? Stop sitting down on the job and get to work yourself. Open communication—take tapes to listen to in the doctor's office."

About the second drawing Dr. Siegel wrote back, "When with family, life is fuller, but trailer is in precarious position. You are all apart…There is more life, color, etc., with family but make sure there is open sharing. And, what are they fishing for?"

She ultimately got an opportunity to meet Dr. Siegel when he was in Seattle for a conference, and spoke at a gathering sponsored by Renewal. Meeting Dr. Siegel was an inspirational event for Nancy. That encounter led to even more conviction on her part that she could survive the disease and get well. Nancy had a strong faith, which enabled her to adopt aspects of meditation and visualization that by themselves might have been contrary to her faith upbringing. She developed her own way to roll them into her prayer time and belief system. That effort provided what became a powerful tool for her, especially when combined with the relaxation tapes provided by her psychologist.

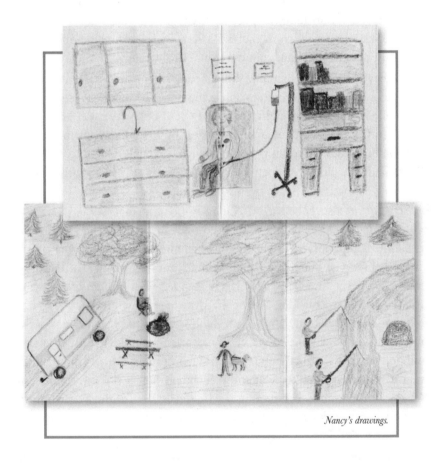

Nancy's drawings.

Father Bob Russell was a young Priest (late 30s) at our church. He was taken aback with the news of Nancy's diagnosis and prognosis and spent a considerable amount of time visiting and praying with Nancy and our whole family. Nancy's outgoing personality had impressed and touched Fr. Bob early on in his young ministry. He appeared a little lost dealing with such a large issue now, possibly the first cancer case of such gravity in his career. His visits were very special. Nancy looked forward to every visit as Fr. Bob was a wonderful nurturer. Besides that I believe Nancy also was providing him with instruction. At the seminary he probably had not received instruction on how we as humans face death. He may not have learned how a young priest could minister to that challenge.

Throughout the chemotherapy treatment regimen, there were some good reports mixed in with some not so good. The oncologist was always upbeat. I believe he truly was encouraged when it appeared the treatments were having a positive effect. The evidence was indirect: there were no new tumors. And for the most part, the malignancies she had were not growing or at least not growing fast. Nancy appeared to tolerate the chemo quite well except for the vomiting and her hair loss. The vomiting was a side effect she hated, especially with the onset of each new treatment regimen, and there were several of those. Nancy was determined to go through each one, and did.

This was an especially horrific process for the rest of the family to be a part of. We all wanted her to stop the treatments at one time or another because they made her so sick. Anti-nausea medications had little effect. At one of her visits with the oncologist, Nancy asked where the cancer would go if it were to spread to another location, other than the spine. The oncologist told her it was common for lung cancer to spread to the brain. Nancy later told me privately that if the cancer did show up in her brain, she wouldn't fight the battle any more. On this issue it didn't matter to her that radiation therapy was often quite effective at shrinking tumors in brain tissue. With pain from the cancer in her spine becoming more of a problem, the oncologist wanted Nancy to have additional radiation treatments. They proved somewhat effective in making it easier for her to lie down, but this second time was not as effective as the first go round.

This experience with cancer had become for all of us a new way of living. It had a lot of rough places and unknowns were always just around the corner. Nancy showed the two children and me her remarkable, determined self. She had this wonderful feistiness and incredible desire to live because she wasn't ready to die. We met and got involved with Renewal, a family of very deep loving affection. The group was always there. Nancy met and developed relationships with several additional medical professionals who spoke at Renewal. All of those people had a positive effect on her journey. We would not have learned about them were it not for Renewal and the passionate leadership of a compassionate Dr. DeShazo.

Nancy's illness also became a challenge for many neighbors and friends. They rose to the occasion because of her need. They did this for someone whom they loved and in spite of knowing she likely would die. Certainly this was also a tough time for our family. Both Nancy and I were concerned about the children. They had become very much aware of what their mother was dealing with. Early on we made the decision to keep them informed as to what was happening, about her treatments, the outlook, etc. Both of them were aware of the initial prognosis. After every doctor appointment when evaluations were made and markers checked whether they showed some change, be it positive or not, the children were given an honest appraisal. This wasn't easy, but we believed it was the right thing to do. They asked their questions; together we often shed our tears.

Nancy was not fond of animals in the house. The children were growing and expressed their desire to have a pet dog. Nancy's brother made financial arrangements with a neighbor whose dog was having a litter to purchase Raphael as a surprise for Nancy. This did not go over well with Nancy. For years Raphael had a rough time living in Nancy's house. He was not allowed on any furniture, especially any of the beds. This picture

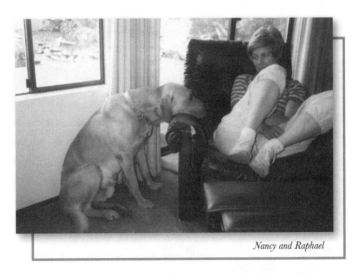

Nancy and Raphael

was taken when Nancy was dealing with the illness. It is in a recliner where they seem to be finally bonding. As the disease ran its course Raphael was usually with Nancy. I have another picture when Nancy, who found it hard to sleep due to the discomfort caused by the tumor in her spine, made her bed on a floor mat with Raphael. Bonding appears to be completed.

Irony or Providence? Nancy was diagnosed in September, 1986. The prognosis given was that she shouldn't expect to live more than 6 months. She discovered Renewal shortly after the diagnosis and became a regular, attending meetings and other functions. Our family had an opportunity to go to Connecticut for a special July 4th celebration. Nancy could not go but insisted the children and I go, so we did. While there, Nancy said in a phone conversation that she was having pain at the base of her skull. When we returned, a brain scan confirmed the cancer had found its way there. Nancy died a month later. Fr. Russell, the priest, who had become very important in Nancy's life, was himself diagnosed with an aggressive leukemia. Due to his own treatments, he was unable to visit with Nancy the last few months of her life and she missed him. He died two weeks before Nancy. She died in August, 1989, almost exactly three years after the diagnosis.

Postscript. Nancy died 20 years ago. That has been so long ago and so much has happened I have added this postscript to fill in the intervening years.

Nancy was a lovingly unique wife and mother. She played a big part in the lives of her family and many of her friends. She was also a great teacher and many of us, including me, learned an immense amount accompanying her during these experiences. There were many disappointments but there also was growth. In early 1991, I found myself in Dr. DeShazo's office. I cannot recall the reason I was there. As I was about to leave Dr. DeShazo asked if I were going to attend the formal opening of the new inpatient hospice center. The Renewal meetings had moved to a conference room there even before the construction was completed, so I knew the place. I remember saying I had been thinking about it but hadn't decided. It came to mind that indeed, I had been thinking about it. Hospice care had already begun even without the inpatient building, and then continued with a shakedown use of the inpatient facility even before the formal opening. Assistance from a hospice team had allowed me to care for Nancy at the end of her illness. When Nancy died she was able to be at home and that is what she wanted. She was in a comfortable and familiar environment, and at peace with everything.

I was with her at the moment of her death. In that moment I felt we both were in the presence of God. Looking back, it was the privilege and experience of caring for Nancy that prepared and encouraged me to want to know more about hospice. So when I told Dr. DeShazo that day I was thinking about attending, he responded with words that still resonate, "I think you should be involved in hospice."

I remember telling him I had been waiting for someone to say just that. I did attend the hospice dedication event. Not long after that Dr. DeShazo had the volunteer coordinator contact me. What happened after that has been an unanticipated continuation of what began when Nancy got sick. It has made for a wonderful journey. It has filled my life with a profound joy that continues still.

After training as a volunteer at the hospice inpatient center, I became an active participant there. After that I started working with the home care division that provided hospice care in patients' homes. Hospice care is centered on providing specialized care for individuals and their loved ones during the final stages in a life-threatening illness. Often it is referred to as comfort care because it takes over after the active treatment focused on cure or stabilization of a chronic illness ends. Hospice care typically is provided during the last six to twelve months of life. That period usually ends in what we call the holy hour of a person's life. It is the most reward-ing work I have ever done. I didn't know it, but caring for Nancy during those three years and especially her last three months, gave me a good understanding of what to expect. Caring for her also revealed that I had a caregiver's heart. I came to believe I was fit to do this very difficult work and I came to love it.

It was while working at the center that I met the inpatient nursing supervisor. Her name was Kay. I began working with her and the other hospice nurses there on a regular basis. After a couple of years Kay and I began dating. Five years after Nancy's death we were married. Yes, God does work in amazing ways, certainly beyond my ability to comprehend.

Several years later Kay and I were invited to join the steering commit-tee for the formation of an all volunteer hospice in the Pacific Northwest. We subsequently took leadership roles in the fledging organization, putting together training and other materials. Our goal was to teach others about coordinating care for patients and their families. Once our program was in place we conducted training for hospice volunteers, drawing the volunteers from the Christian church community. We trained our students in the same methods used to equip lay Stephen Ministers in churches, modifying materials for end of life and bereavement care. The organization has worked well within the church community and with various hospice organizations in the area.

So, life goes on. A once-promising, loving relationship with Nancy and our children seemed to end tragically with her diagnosis and untimely death. Our lives were upended but that has been replaced with another wonderful relationship with Kay. After what we went through together I have a much greater appreciation for life and living. I also have a new understanding of death and dying. I feel I continue to grow and learn in every possible way, especially spiritually. What changed in the middle of my life was made possible only through Nancy's end of life experience. Both of our children have also grown and now are married and have their own families. Each child worked through the loss of their mom in different ways and that process continues even today. Nancy will always be a big part of all of our lives.

— Rose and John —

Rose wrote this story herself at my request. She and John moved away to an arid mountain community after he retired. They are both doing well and divide their time between travel, visiting their grandchildren and other family, and making their own wine. So this is Rose writing about her experience.

I want to tell you first about my cancer treatment. I took pride that I always kept my yearly gynecological and mammogram appointments. At age 47, some four or five months after my last such appointment, I felt a lump in my left breast as I was drying off after a shower. Of course, I was scared.

I had grown up with a huge fear of cancer. There was a lot of cancer in my mother's French-Canadian family. Her father had died of colon cancer at age 47 in 1928. My mother herself had four types of cancer and survived all of them. Her sister had, and survived, three types. Mother's brother died of esophageal cancer when he was 42. My youngest brother had colon cancer at 32 and survived it. No one, however, had ever had breast cancer.

I immediately made an appointment with my gynecologist. He said he also could feel the lump. He referred me to Dr. DeShazo. Dr. DeShazo seemed very kind. He said he would do a needle biopsy as it was possible this lump was just a cyst. I was nervous and scared as he did the biopsy. I was to come back to hear the results of the biopsy in a week.

When I came back a week later John, my husband, came with me to the appointment. We were told the biopsy showed malignancy. I totally fell apart. I was lucky John was there because I'm sure I only heard a fraction of what the doctor was saying. I was stunned. Why me? This isn't fair! What will I do? Will I be able to see my son graduate from high school in June—two months away? Will I see my two children marry? Will I ever see grandchildren? What will John do?

John asked the doctor about statistics and how best for us to decide what to do. The doctor told us to try and live in the moment—one day at a time—and that was how we would figure out what was best for me. He also recommended a book by Dr. Bernie Siegel, *Love, Medicine, and Miracles*.

We were able to get that and several other books about cancer at the library. I immediately started in reading them all. There was a message of hope in them, especially in Dr. Siegel's book.

My surgery was scheduled for April 11, 1990. I had several weeks to wait while all the testing was done so I got on the phone with the local hospitals and found that a nearby hospital had a breast cancer support group. I attended a meeting before my surgery. There I met women who had been through what I was approaching. I was amazed that one woman was a ten year survivor! Some group members gave me their phone numbers and invited me to call them if I had questions. I felt supported and felt I had a little more information to work with. Those women told me about the strange drain I would be going home from the hospital with. During this time Dr. DeShazo sent John and me to discuss options with several other specialists. He thought we might want to hear from others what to expect.

The radiation oncologist spent several hours with us. He was very kind and thorough in his explanation and the drawings he made. The medical oncologist I saw also was informative. He was very low-key but answered all our questions. He had a nice nurse who was also very helpful. It turned out she was also a breast cancer survivor.

Then there was the plastic surgeon who talked to me about reconstruction at the time of my mastectomy. After talking to him and seeing the pictures, I decided that to me, the pictures didn't look that good. Plus, I didn't like the idea of having the silicone implants, which they were using at that time, in my body. This just wasn't me. Knowing I could change my mind and have reconstruction anytime later, I decided not to do it.

The night before my surgery we decided to take the advice of our good friend, Sue Geary, a nurse. We went out to dinner at one of our favorite restaurants. The food was wonderful, but I felt like I was in a dream. Was all this really happening?

Finally April 11 arrived. I was admitted. My nurse friend, Sue, came to make sure I was comfortable, even though she wasn't assigned to that floor. She got me an egg crate foam mat for my bed. Diane and Joe, my two college age children, were there to wait with John.

I was prepped for the mastectomy. I was able to bring a walkman and headphones so I could be listening to nice music during surgery—another Bernie Siegel idea. Dr. DeShazo, my surgeon, was OK with this.

The next thing I remember is that I was in the recovery room and the doctor said I did well. I stayed in the hospital two days. John and the kids were frequent visitors. My son Joe, almost 18, showed up one day in a loud Hawaiian shirt he had picked up at a local thrift store. He bought that outrageous shirt because he heard laughter accelerated healing. Diane, who was 20, had written a beautiful Palanca letter to me before my operation that made me feel so loved and appreciated.

When Dr. DeShazo discharged me he said to come to his office in a week to hear the pathology report. So, I went home with that little drain in place, just like the support group ladies had told me about. At home, recovery went well. My son Joe gave me a big dowel rod to use to tap on the floor to summon him from downstairs if I needed anything. It wasn't very high tech but it worked for us. The next week the news about the pathology report was good. No lymph nodes were involved. Dr. DeShazo thought I would just need to take tamoxifen, an estrogen blocker, because the tumor was estrogen receptor positive. Dr. DeShazo mentioned that he had a support group for all types of cancer patients called Renewal. It met once a week at the hospital where I had the surgery. He invited me to come to the Group.

He also had me go back to the medical oncologist to get a second opinion. The oncologist said my tumor was an aggressive one. So, even though I didn't have lymph node involvement, he recommended CMF chemotherapy (that's Cytoxin, methotrexate, and 5-FU) for nine months. He told me my hair probably would not fall out but it might become thin. This idea of taking chemo was a surprise. Having to make these decisions without knowing much was quite difficult for me. John was glad, however, that I didn't have to have radiation as he has a real thing against it.

So, it was time to make a decision. I finally reached the conclusion that I had to do everything in my power to fight this. So I went for the chemo. I tolerated CMF well at first. But, after a few months, I would be sick the night I had the treatment, then OK the rest of the three weeks until the next dose. They didn't have all the anti-nausea medicines then that they do today. The nine months passed and then I started on tamoxifen which I took for an additional five years. I didn't have any problems with that.

I had to have checkups. They came often at first. Now, it's 18 years later and I'm back to the yearly mammogram. I am scared every time, but life goes on. Those two college aged kids are both married now and I have three wonderful grandchildren. God has been good to me.

I mentioned attending a breast cancer group at another hospital. After a year or so there a group of us started a similar group at our own hospital. The group was called Bosom Buddies and it was just for women breast cancer survivors. So, I had two groups to go to. I liked Bosom Buddies. It also met close to my house and met during the day, which I liked. We were all about the same age and seemed to have a lot in common. We were all fighting the same disease and had unique insights into the drugs like tamoxifen and other problems like swelling of the arm [lymphedema], hot flashes and chemo brain.

I formed close bonds with many of these women, just like I did at Renewal. Several times the women's group went off to Lake Quinault for a fun weekend. We stayed at a member's cabin. We marched together in Race for the Cure and Relay for Life. We enjoyed going out to lunch after our meetings. I still keep in touch with some of those women even though I have moved away.

Two years ago I was diagnosed with endometrial cancer. There weren't many symptoms with this, other than a tiny amount of spotting. After a uterine biopsy showed a very aggressive tumor, the local gynecologist where I live sent me to Seattle to the Seattle Cancer Care Alliance. I had a complete hysterectomy at the University of Washington Hospital by a Gyn surgical oncologist. I was in the University hospital three days. The pathology report didn't show any lymph node involvement so I was told to have an exam and pap smear every three months. I did that for a year and a half. Now I'm on a six month schedule. I divide my appointments between the doctor at the Cancer Alliance and my local gynecologist.

About Renewal: Dr. DeShazo suggested I attend his support group. I decided to give it a try. It met on Monday afternoons at four p.m. in a meeting room at the hospital. There were 20-30 people there who were survivors of many types of cancer. They had a great library. You could borrow the books. A nice gentleman, George W., spoke to me the first time I walked in. He was very welcoming. Dr. DeShazo was the leader but everyone got a chance to talk.

So I started attending regularly. A wide variety of things happened at Renewal. Sometimes we had speakers. We had a dream therapist. We had an Ayurvedic doctor. We had a naturopath. There was a psychologist who taught us to do guided imagery. We had a course on Tai chi. We even smoked a Native American pipe. We made kumbacha tea. Dr. DeShazo and the whole group seemed open to whatever works.

Gerri Haynes, the first director of the Community Hospice was always full of wisdom. She often came to Renewal and led the discussions. Because of her, several of us took the training and became hospice volunteers. I took the training in 1990 and from 1991 until we moved away in 2002, I was a hospice volunteer. That was a very enlightening and rewarding experience for me.

One memorable woman who came to the group, Pam D., had a brain tumor at one time. She told us how her tumor shrank because she visualized it getting smaller and smaller until it disappeared.

Renewal was always ready for a party. The Halloween parties were the

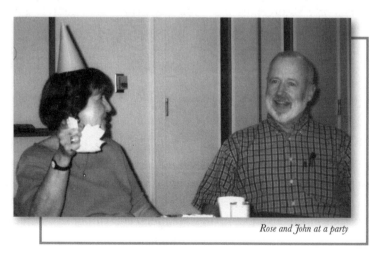

Rose and John at a party

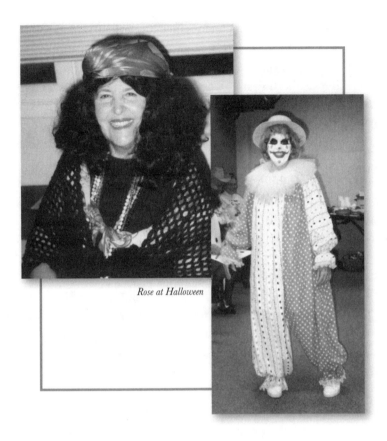

Rose at Halloween

best. Most people dressed up. Dr. DeShazo always had great costumes. He came once dressed as a logger, another time an apple-picker, another time a nun. His wife Maureen used to come and bring their children. Their kids did a "chicken dance" for us at one of the parties.

The group had several other memorable members. Trude was one. She was always so supportive and fun to be around. She dazzled us with stories of visiting her native Germany and going to spas for healing. She showed us her method of packing her small suitcase and traveler's vest with everything she needed for an extended stay.

John Barnett was, and is, amazing. He keeps very busy helping others. He found time to write his own book on aging. He started a support group for prostate cancer at the University of Washington. He took us on a field trip to the arboretum and performed a tea ceremony for us. He still manages to get some of us together to have lunch every once in a while.

Pat W. and Fran P. were always there with a smile and encouragement. Cathy W. and her husband George were some of the party planners. Donna and Wayne T. took over the party detail in later years. They, along with Margaret and Paul F. were all devoted to each other and to all of us. Margaret P. was struggling with leukemia. She decided to have a bone marrow transplant. Her courage was so inspiring. She told us about the East West bookstore and her experience with a healer she used to telephone in another state. Nancy K., another of our members, had an amazing way of leading us through guided imagery. She was very inspiring. One of Dr. DeShazo's most memorable statements to all of us was, "When you wake up in the morning ask yourself, what fun thing will I do today?" That should be the one thing you should be sure to do.

I think I'm giving you the idea that lots of new ideas and possibilities surfaced at Renewal. I had never been one to go for a lot of unorthodox ideas. But with the support of the rest of the group, I had the courage to try.

I had acupuncture several times from Clara, a naturopath who was John Barnett's daughter. It was amazing and very relaxing. I tried the telephone healer too, but wasn't convinced of any benefits from that.

Our members all grew close to one another. We were like family. We heard about each others' families, the weddings, the births. Sometimes we attended funerals of our members as a group. The group was there for me. Two years ago, just before I had the surgery for endometrial cancer, I received calls, cards, visits, and a lot of loving support. Happy or sad, we were fighting cancer together.

I want everyone to know that my husband John was there with me when I received the devastating news I had breast cancer. He came to all my important appointments with me. He had good questions for the doctors—things I hadn't thought of. He's still always there for me. He knows how to reassure me.

John made a meditation tape for me to listen to when I had chemo. It had Pacabel's Canon in D playing in the background along with John's soothing voice giving me assurance. After my first chemo John took me to an upscale local market for some fresh squeezed juice. He had read that beet and celery juice were good for you.

John would come to the Renewal parties after work. He'd share our potlucks and get to see all my friends. He learned how to give back rubs from a library video. Those back rubs were wonderful and helped me feel much better. He became really interested. He went on to school and became a licensed massage practitioner.

Every year on the anniversary of my breast cancer surgery we celebrate survivorship by going out to lunch or a special dinner. After our son and daughter finished college we were able to take some trips. We especially loved our trip to Italy and visiting the home town of my immigrant grandparents near Bari.

John is always reading about vitamins and always makes sure I take the latest ones he thinks are best for me. I'm lucky to have John as my helpmate. I doubt there are many men who are so loving and supportive.

— Margaret and Paul —

(This is Margaret F. in distinction to the story of Margaret P. in Chapter 2.) Margaret is a good example of how a person's story can play out differently from what they are told to prepare for. Margaret had what she still describes as an ideal life. For most of their professional lives she and her husband lived in various places in the Middle East. Paul worked for oil companies. Margaret was a registered nurse and able to work in a variety of roles and capacities. The two of them did this so that they could be together, travel together for all those exotic experiences, and also be able to raise their daughter together. They moved back from their last posting in Dubai in 1985. Margaret was 65 years old and the couple had decided to retire in the Pacific Northwest. During this transition Margaret began thinking she felt a lump in her left breast, but three different doctors she saw could not find it. Finally she was referred to a surgeon. He did locate the lump and took it out in 1987. It was a malignancy and he wanted to do a mastectomy. Margaret elected to have just a lumpectomy and node dissection. The pathology report said the nodes were negative for metastases. She followed the surgery with a course of radiation but chemotherapy was deemed not necessary.

Within a year of that original surgery Margaret developed three growths on her forehead. She called them her "bumps." One was biopsied. She was told the one removed and the two remaining all represented spread from her breast cancer. She was advised (or elected, she doesn't remember which) not to have any more treatment since she was told the prognosis was poor and she did not have very long to live. One of the practitioners she saw told her she should find a support group. This initial treatment was done in Oregon but after that she and Paul decided to settle in adjacent Washington. About a year after that her inquiries led her to the Renewal group.

In the years that followed Margaret and Paul were regulars at the weekly Renewal meetings. She was resigned to the poor prognosis she had been given. She told the group that she viewed the "bumps" on her forehead as reminders each morning when she looked in the mirror that she should make the most out of the day ahead, as time might be short.

Paul proved to be an example of what a support person can mean to someone with cancer. Margaret, by her own admission, has always tended to view events negatively. Paul was just the opposite. He had a wonderful sense of humor and helped balance her negativity. He could generally be counted on for a humorous anecdote or joke at our weekly meetings. And so the group, and the two of them, went along like this for years.

Then, in one of life's ironies, Paul had an unanticipated and fatal heart

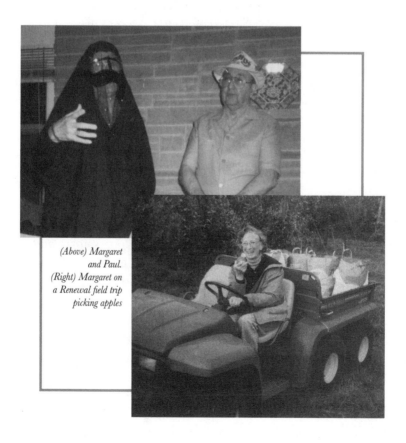

(Above) Margaret and Paul. (Right) Margaret on a Renewal field trip picking apples

attack in 1997. He had never had any symptoms of heart disease. Margaret remembers it was all over within 30 minutes. In the years that followed Margaret continued to attend our meetings regularly, either by herself or with her daughter. She developed other medical problems, notably osteoporosis and kyphosis (a hump in the back due to osteoporosis and collapse of the vertebra). She also developed a bothersome sensitivity to cold in her finger tips (Reynaud's phenomenon). She had to start using a cane and sometimes a walker but was determined to remain active. She could never abide sitting around watching television. She began going to the local senior center to find activities to keep her busy. Margaret is now 89. That trouble in 1987 is a distant memory. A typical week now includes her regular German lessons (she always wanted to learn the language), knitting and crocheting circles, and a separate day of attending a craft group.

The "bumps" on her forehead remained until 2004. She developed a separate, serious skin cancer, a basal cell carcinoma, at the edge of her left nostril. An extensive resection that went down into the oral cavity was required, but the plastic surgeon that performed the procedure did a good, complete, job. At my suggestion she got the surgeon to remove her two forehead bumps at the same time. And yes, both were consistent with the metastatic breast cancer as had been diagnosed 16 years before. For whatever reason, those early metastases which led to dire predictions about her future were the extent of it. The original cancer still has never spread any further.

— George and Cathy —

George was a patient in the mid 1980s after he retired as a truck driver for one of the major oil companies. He was a lifelong smoker and, about six months after retirement, he started coughing up blood. He was found to have lung cancer. The cancer was extensive and at surgery I had to remove his entire left lung.

George was another tough, no-nonsense type of guy. Over a period of months as we got to know each other better, I found out what an interesting person he was. George was born in 1924. Like many men from that period much of his life was defined by what he did in WWII. When I congratulated him upon how well he had handled the lung cancer episode he responded by saying he hadn't worried about it, or anything else for that matter. George felt that since the war every day had been given to him as a gift.

George had been a naval aviator flying a Corsair off an aircraft carrier. He related to me the story about how he had been shot down by the Japanese in 1944. This came out in a piecemeal fashion, one little anecdote at a time. His plane was hit and he crashed. He was left floating in the Pacific alone for nine days until finally being discovered and rescued. He survived on the raw fish he caught and rain water. He almost died in several close calls with sharks. He told me he went from a pre-crash weight of about 170 to 90 pounds by the time he was pulled out and taken to recover in a hospital. He did recover and was able to rejoin his squadron at war's end. He and the rest of his unit sailed back on the carrier to San Francisco.

He told me how it was customary for all aircraft to take off and fly in formation as the flotilla approached the West Coast. "We were going to Mare Island," obviously relishing telling his favorite story once again, "and the only thing the skipper passed along was that we were supposed to stay in formation. Absolutely no one was to break formation until the approach for landing. And to fly under the Golden Gate Bridge—that was verboten!"

Well, George in his exuberance about his recent rescue did break formation. He dove and flew under the Golden Gate. As far as he knew, he was the only one to disobey orders. "After I landed I got called to the commander's office right away." George continued, "He chewed me out and asked why I did it. I told him, just for the hell of it! He told me he should put me in the brig but he just busted me back to ensign and let me go."

Right after he was discharged, George and Cathy married and had one son. George worked for Standard Oil of California for 43 years, ending up as a supervisor. By his standards George felt he had a pretty tame life and he enjoyed all of it. He loved collecting cars and bowling and playing golf. He had an Edsel among his vehicles, but his pride was a Buick Riviera with the big 425 cubic inch engine. After retirement the couple had moved back to Washington State and that's how he wound up coming to see me.

After the lung cancer surgery George and Cathy started coming to Renewal. He felt comfortable talking to me about the stuff in the Navy because I had been in the Navy and been to Vietnam. At Renewal George joined in the discussions from the point of view of a man old enough to know a lot about life. Cathy enjoyed talking about her Welsh ancestry and growing up in eastern Washington. George was happy to let Cathy do the research on what life changes they needed to make. Both of them got interested in Native American healing rituals and lore. They went shopping and exploring for what they could find about such mysteries and brought new ideas they discovered to share with the group. They both enjoyed talking to everyone and kept our phone tree up to date. They took responsibility for helping prepare our parties and potluck meals and were our chief gift buyers.

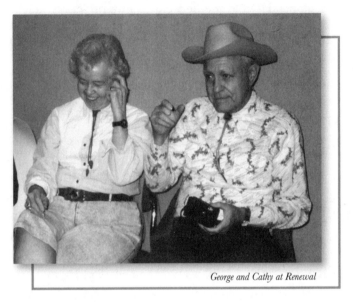

George and Cathy at Renewal

A couple of years later George had rectal bleeding and was found to have colon cancer. He came back to me to have a portion of his colon removed. That whole episode also left George unphased and he continued life as before. A couple of years after that he developed a much more serious problem: a tumor appeared on his left chest wall and started growing rapidly. This was about six years after his lung cancer and defied any attempts to control it. In my private conversations with him George seemed to realize that his time was up and this was the one that would get him. In various ways he expressed that he had had a good run. He continued to talk mostly about the quiet practical things of everyday life and continued with his hobbies. He died August 17, 1993 at age 69.

Cathy continued coming to Renewal. The friends she and George had made there were a real source of support to her. She continued with her customary activities in the group. In 1998 Cathy was diagnosed with breast cancer. She had a lumpectomy and radiation and felt comfortable that was enough treatment for her. This new health problem of her own caused her to shift to new interests among the women talking about breast cancer. She stayed in the house she and George had made their home. Her son lived nearby and gave his mother a lot of support such as taking her to church on Sunday with his family. Whenever possible Cathy drove herself to our meetings and whereever she needed to go. She drove the streets in that same canary yellow Buick Riviera, just like George had done. She continued these activities until she had to move to an assisted living facility for her last year. She died peacefully at age 84.

— Wayne and Donna —

This couple had a story somewhat similar to George and Cathy although Wayne had been in the Army in Korea. They too were an older couple living in retirement and needing to adapt to the changes cancer made in their lives. Wayne and Donna lived in a small village about 20 miles east of the metropolitan area and drove their Jeep in every week for the meetings. Wayne had been a smoker since 1929 and developed lung cancer. Another local surgeon had removed Wayne's left lung in 1992. He was told the procedure was definitive and that no other treatment would be necessary. Shortly after that the couple found out about Renewal and started attending faithfully.

Wayne had been a pharmacist in the Army during the Korean War. This background led to quite an interest in nutritional supplements. He was always investigating things he could take to strengthen his immune system and Donna was always there to support him. Wayne's comments usually were based upon something he had learned as he researched new ideas. Together they tended a large garden at home and grew almost all their food. Donna was very creative about cooking and preserving food. She either preserved or froze what they grew and that was most of what they ate. She became a model of practicality among the more abstract discussions about organic foods and natural ways of doing things. She was also very creative and made many things at home. These crafts came to Renewal and were displayed from time to time. Donna became the principal organizer of the menu and decorations for our potluck meals and themed celebrations.

Our Halloween parties were always very special and highly competitive affairs. Costumes were sometimes ornate and often very clever. The first Halloween Wayne and Donna attended the group they entered, both under a white bed sheet with two points pinched above their heads. Green paint was on the side of the sheet, everywhere except on these two highest points. Guessing what everyone else's disguise represented was part of the fun but we were stumped by Wayne and Donna's costume. When we all gave up, the two of them under the sheet raised their arms gleefully and shouted the answer, "Twin Peaks!" Maybe I would have gotten it if I had been watching more television in the early 1990s. Wayne and Donna won

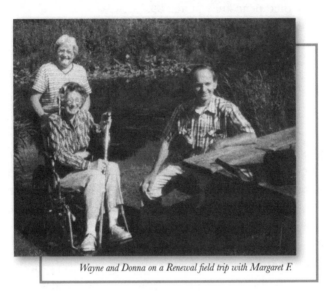

Wayne and Donna on a Renewal field trip with Margaret F.

the Best Costume award that year.

Almost exactly ten years after his surgery Wayne started having pain in the back of his neck. He turned out to have a late recurrence of his lung cancer in his upper thoracic spine. Over the next year he gradually grew weaker while receiving radiation treatment at the local VA hospital. Making the drive in to our meetings finally became too uncomfortable. A couple of times the group went out to Wayne's home and visited the couple just so we could see him again. Especially during that last year Donna continued to care for him so he could stay at home and in his special easy chair until the end. He finally died on December 30, 2003. He was 80 years old.

When I talked to Donna in 2007 and 2008 about their experience at Renewal she had many good memories. "Being with so many different people was a whole new experience for us," she began. "There were new things we had never heard about, and Wayne really liked that." She felt they had been in a very small circle of friends out in the country where they lived. Coming to the meetings really expanded their world. "With so many things to think about," she continued, "hearing what was said at Renewal really settled us down about what to do. It helped us so much. I really think it helped Wayne make peace with everything.

"Wayne believed very much in mind over matter," she went on. "So Renewal gave him a lot of reinforcement. For a long time we were sure things were working for him." She tended to downplay the great help she provided in keeping the meeting activities running smoothly each week. It was as if she felt her efforts were payback for the benefit of knowledge and socialization they received.

Donna kept her own book identifying the people she met at Renewal and what they said about their self-help activities. "At first I didn't want to hear all those stories about cancer," she said. "Then I came around. There was something very good for both of us about being there."

— Gloria and John —

The story of this couple is one I want to relate for a couple of reasons. Gloria had breast cancer and I operated on her. Maybe it is enough to say that her husband John just worshipped her. It was quite something to see the tenderness and almost furtive affection they shared. They were in their fifties when we all met. She was small in stature and scared to death of cancer and everything that came with it.

John was a big man. Maybe a bit overweight, but physically one of those burly, fast-moving men whose size makes you want to get out of the way. You could tell he was frustrated that his partner was burdened with cancer, and somehow he couldn't find the right instrument to get it off of her. He worked with her to sort out the recommendations for treatment. He explained everything to her and supported her, but all along he appeared to be looking for an opportunity. If he could just find some way to get hold of this cancer thing, to crush it in his big hands, to smash it…then everything in their life could go back to being normal. So they too made a good balance like some of our other couples. John pushing ahead, wanting to know what the hell all this means and ready to make decisions. And Gloria, at his side but trailing a little, cautious and usually wanting to put things off, somewhat embarrassed. But you could see she was very glad her

John was up front, running interference.

They came to Renewal in the 1980s after Gloria's treatment had ended. They participated fully and were a real asset to the group. Renewal was not an intellectual pursuit for Gloria and John. They were there to be with other people like themselves, commiserate about their troubles, learn a few things, but mostly to go on with life as they wanted.

The two of them had several uneventful years, then Gloria had a recurrence. She had metastases to her lung that were diffuse and beyond any hope of surgery. She was started on chemotherapy and it made her very sick. Her apprehension was terrible. John was always there, taking care of her in his tender way. The other side of him, usually held in check, was thinking somebody had to be responsible for this. If John could just figure out who, he'd smash him. The disease progressed. Gloria developed an effusion or fluid build-up around her lungs. It was much worse on one side than the other. Gloria started seeing a pulmonary specialist so I lost track of her for a while.

Then I got a call from John. Gloria had gone back to the pulmonary specialist to have fluid drained from around her lung. The fluid was compressing her lungs and causing difficulty breathing and anxiety. John reported, as soon as the pulmonologist had put a needle to her chest, Gloria had collapsed. She fainted and fell on the floor. John wanted me to take over. When I telephoned that doctor to hear what he had to say, he had been spooked by the whole thing. He said he would be glad if I took over.

So later that day I met Gloria and John. As a precaution I arranged for the meeting to be in the emergency room of our hospital. The emergency room was all set up in case anything bad happened and it was convenient. It was, however, an impersonal place for the three of us to have a serious discussion. I looked at her x-rays. One lung had "white out" or opacity due to that side of the chest being so full of fluid.

I turned back to the two of them there in the treatment room. By now Gloria was in a gown, sitting on a gurney, with all the apparatus there for me to do a needle aspiration. "How do you feel?" I asked. "How do you feel about my draining off the fluid?"

Gloria was very anxious, "Okay, I guess." She hesitated again, "It really isn't too bad, though, the breathing, I mean. It's not so bad."

I could feel John's tightening up even though he was several feet from me. He wound even tighter because he wanted to interrupt and contradict her. But he didn't. He didn't say anything. He just wanted her to be well. These several years of living with this thing, this goddamned breast cancer, as he called it, had really taken its toll on both of them. Despite their anxiousness, I felt confident they both trusted me. They were willing to do anything I suggested and at the moment I didn't see any big rush. Gloria had already had a hard day.

"Well," I ventured, "if you aren't having too much trouble right now, why don't we wait?" What I said was more of a psychological judgment than a clinical one. I was concerned that she was strung out. If I tried to puncture her chest and she fainted again, that would be bad. "Why don't we wait a day or two before deciding? We can always do this later."

Gloria nodded. That was just fine. She turned to John with a "let's go!" look. He hesitated for a moment and then agreed. John helped her out to their car and they went home.

Gloria died about a week later. John came to Renewal and said she had died at home over the weekend. Despite all the breathing trouble it had been fairly peaceful. She had just faded away, her protector beside her. John came to talk to me after the meeting. He was still John, but the tenseness had deflated. He spoke in a matter-of-fact way and thanked me for all I had done and tried to do. That was nice to hear, and I responded with something equally complimentary, but what John said next was far more instructive and always has stayed with me. It became a useful reminder how in certain moments every word, or even how words are said, can have a pivotal effect.

"Doc," John said, "I know what you said last week was what you thought was best. Still, when Gloria heard you say you didn't think we needed to draw that fluid out, she took it another way." Grief cracked his voice, "She took it that you thought it didn't make any difference what we did." He paused for long seconds composing himself, "That it wouldn't do any good. She went home thinking you were telling her it must finally be all over."

My first impulse was to say something. I wanted to say that had not been my intention...but I kept silent.

John didn't expect an answer anyway. Gloria was gone and things like funeral arrangements needed his attention. John put a consoling hand on my shoulder then impulsively pulled me into a bear hug. She was gone now. He was alone and there was no answer.

This next part about John is a little more lively and upbeat. John kept coming to Renewal for a number of months. I can't remember if he told us or we just heard from someone, John became friends with Gloria's best friend. This was a woman neighbor who had come in and helped care for Gloria in those last months. About a year after Gloria died we heard that this woman and John had gotten married. He had stopped coming to Renewal and then they were gone.

Gloria died in 1990. John left in 1991. In 2001 he came back. One day, after a Renewal meeting had already started, John just walked in and gave me a wave. Quite a few of the people there didn't know who this late arrival was. I remembered him, of course, and think I said, "John! Where the hell have you been?"

"Traveling," was the reply. John took a seat and looked around the circle for faces he might know. "After Gloria died, I had nothing to keep me here. I sold the house. Got rid of everything. I got married again and we bought a big motor home. Decided to go on the road and see the country." John then went on to tell an attentive audience how he mapped out a big circular route around the USA. He and the new wife started out, driving all the way to Florida via the northern tier of states. Then they came back across the southwest and up through California. It had taken them a couple of years. After that they started moving back and forth or up and down. They stayed in places like Montana in the summer and went back to Arizona and the Southwest in the winter. "We made a lot of friends, you know? You see the same people. You get to know them after a few times. You say to them up in Montana, 'See you in such-and-such a trailer park in Arizona.' And next time you go, they're there!"

After listening I was curious to know why John had returned.

John was ready with his answer. It was clear he enjoyed being back, telling this tale, but he became a bit more somber in his reply, "We decided to sell the motor home and come back to Seattle to settle down. Too dangerous," he made a dismissive swing outward with one arm. "Too many old folks out there." He concluded adding, "I was sixty when we drove out of Seattle. It's ten years later and now I'm seventy…and we were some of the young ones! It's too scary. There are old guys a lot older than me on the road now. They've gotten too old and don't know it. Old guys in motor homes big as trucks. Some of them can't hear, can't see, too weak to change a tire if they have a flat. Too dangerous being out there…I'm staying off the road from now on."

CHAPTER 4

RENEWED:
INFLUENCE AND HAVING AN EFFECT

— John Barnett —

John is an example of a Renewal member who handled his own medical problems (prostate cancer) then accepted new challenges. He has learned how to build upon personal experiences to help others. He was the first group member to start his own cancer support group, then he wrote a book. John has moved on, seeing a way to influence the political process. I asked John to write this chapter explaining what influenced him and the evolution of his thought.

En route to learn the result of my biopsy I was confident that the doctor would convey a clean bill of health. The reason? I was merely being a good citizen by volunteering for the male blood draw for prostate research being done at the University. There were never any symptoms of a problem. Anyway, just two months earlier a specialist had told me that I did not have to worry about that particular kind of cancer.

It was a shock, therefore, when the doctor, a complete stranger to me, looked me in the eye and said, "I am sorry to tell you Mr. Barnett, you do have prostate cancer." The ride back home from the hospital was terrible. I drove alone and pondered how this would change my future life. And, indeed, would my life be shortened? I recalled that all four of my grandparents had died in their 60s – of cancer. Our last child was still a teenager.

Would the possibility of my early death affect her future adversely? I shall never forget that day's lonely drive home.

In somber tones I relayed to my wife what the doctor had said. She, being raised a very private person, said. "Let's not tell anyone for a while." This was just the opposite from my instinctual reaction, which was to shout to the housetops, "I am devastated to suddenly learn that I have cancer. I am afraid that I might die! Can anyone help me?"

It would be a month before I could see the doctor conducting that university research project that discovered my cancer. I had to wait to learn, not patiently, of possible options to extend my life. In the meantime I was antsy to absorb anything I could to provide some knowledge of my disease. Eventually that could help me to arrive at a more informed decision of what course of therapy to pursue, if indeed therapy was available. This was before the days of online research, a time when medical information was not so easy to come by. I was at a loss to know where to turn.

I remembered the American Cancer Society. Wouldn't they want to help me, I wondered. A telephone call to that organization was answered by a volunteer who referred me to a support group, Renewal, which met weekly at a nearby hospital. My desire to begin this terrible education process was stronger than my reluctance to seem vulnerable in front of strangers. I showed up at the next meeting, not knowing what to expect.

A support group was something completely foreign to me. Would I be embarrassed for what I did not know about my condition? I had not yet had a consultation with a doctor other than to learn that cancer was already evident in my body. Would the support experience without first seeing a doctor even be worthwhile? Really, I was less interested in what other cancer sufferers in a support group might have to say and more interested in talking with a doctor as soon as possible. I couldn't know at that time how profoundly Renewal would affect my subsequent life – and that I would still be meeting weekly with the group even thirteen years later.

That day I seated myself in a hospital meeting room among twenty complete strangers.

Soon I felt that the experience might have been worth the trip. The facilitator of the support group, it turned out, was a medical doctor; a person with a soft, pleasant Southern accent. After his brief introduction, participants started giving updates, one-by-one, on the present status of their serious medical conditions. Some had received recent good news and were elated. Others reported pessimistic outcomes and were obviously worried. Some women cried. I made up my mind that, being a man, and despite how I felt inside, it would not serve my self-image to cry. When it came their turn to speak, some simply identified themselves as being there for the support of the spouse or parent who sat beside them.

People testified about their various life-threatening diseases, but mostly cancer. I can't remember learning anything at that meeting that contributed to my scanty knowledge of my particular disease. No one there had had that kind of cancer. What did impress me, however, was the number of people who were willing – even eager – to talk about their very personal health problems. Equally impressive was the fact that all of the listeners, despite their own perilous conditions, listened attentively to each worried word of the speaker.

Not only did they listen but they also gave indications by various nods and comments of their understanding and support of the speaker. Some asked questions of the speaker, which revealed their prior knowledge and memory of what had been reported in earlier meetings. They acted genuinely interested and concerned. Participants rose above their own condition of sorrow to reach out to worried victims of life-threatening diseases. So this is what a support group does, I realized. Perhaps even a man could participate without embarrassment and also get something useful from it.

My turn to speak was short since I had little information about my condition to convey. The medical doctor facilitator, Dr. Claude DeShazo, listened carefully, paused, and then asked some questions for which I had no replies. However, my impression was that when the right time came he would probably be helpful. I foresaw that this could be extremely useful since I knew no other specialists who were experienced at working with cancer patients.

Renewal included features that may be uncommon to other groups. Each session was more than simply a recital of participants' states of bodies and minds. Also included were various elements of education. One was a lending library of five shelves of books, mostly on overcoming cancer. The good doctor himself had bought many volumes, carefully choosing what might be most appropriate and helpful. Users contributed other volumes that they had purchased and found helpful. Family survivors of previous attendees who were no longer in this world donated some.

A volunteer librarian catalogued the collection and reminded us when they were overdue. Motivational books were also included along with audiotapes and videocassettes on thinking positively, and other mental and spiritual aids to combating stress and depression. Someone had recorded audio comedy programs from yesteryear. Laughter, it seems, serves one well when faced with otherwise depressing thoughts. I made frequent use of this library and felt that I was the better for it.

Another education feature was guest speakers who came once a month or more. Specialists in any area that focused on strengthening mind or body were welcomed. The range of subjects was vast. We heard talks, and got to ask questions, on Tai chi, meditation, dream interpretation, Ayurvedic and naturopathic medicine, music as therapy (classic is in; rock, out), aromatherapy, imaging, nutrition, neurolinguistic programming, and many, many more. It was always a treat to look forward to having one's horizons broadened in this way; something you wouldn't normally do for yourself. It was a valuable education, free for attendance. And, yes, it did serve to augment whatever else I was learning from other customary sources. And it did contribute to my overall well-being. One speaker, a medical doctor, so impressed me that I made him my family doctor. That was ten years ago. He continues to impress me to this day.

It wasn't only outside guest speakers from whom we learned useful information. Members of the group shared their time-tested prescriptions for such things as lessening the nausea and fatigue resulting from chemotherapy and radiation. Some of this practical advice would not always be forthcoming even from personal physicians. Probably they themselves had not been victims of a particular disease. Or, they did not take the time to spread what they had learned from their patients. Or, the patient had not asked the important questions. It takes a victim who has had to learn by experimentation to be able to help other victims with what worked for them. One gentleman testified on how a macrobiotic diet had extended his life. (I immediately bought that book.) This learning from each other is one of the strengths of a support group.

Progress toward a cure in an individual Renewal participant was cause for a celebration, as was every notable holiday or festival. Any excuse for a party was enthusiastically supported by the entire group. Occasions were Valentine's Day, Easter, Memorial Day, Independence Day, Labor Day, Thanksgiving, etc. All birthdays were noted in a calendar and celebrated one day per month. Shortly after I joined the group it was announced that Halloween would be feted by a potluck dinner and masquerade party. Not knowing to what extent people dressed, and not wishing to overly stand out with some freakish costume, I arrived with a modest mask and hat. To my surprise, people had gone all out. Many had made their own costumes, some quite elaborate. One couple came as walking crayons. A woman was a geisha.

Despite his or her attempts at concealment I could recognize almost everyone in the group. However, I could not spot our leader, Dr. DeShazo. Nor did I recognize the person in a full nun's black and white habit. On further examination, lo and behold, it was Dr. DeShazo himself! After that I saw him in costumes representing Paul Bunyon, King Solomon, Uncle Sam, and others. Is this doctor for real, I wondered at my first party, or is he a party animal masquerading as a physician? It turned out that he did enjoy partying as well as the rest of us, probably even more so. And, yes, parties are indeed great for putting aside the more serious and sobering cares of daily life for an interlude of laughter and good times. Parties are therapeutic.

And comfort food was plentiful. At every weekly meeting there was something on which to snack. We enjoyed all kinds of herbal teas. You would think that for special parties we would plan in advance what food item each would bring. It never happened. Yet, it always worked out that there would be at least one item of substance along with some vegetables, salads and fruit, and plenty of desserts. One attendant shared her recipe for homemade pickled vegetables, which had been a big hit with everyone. Indeed, food is comforting.

Gatherings were not always held indoors. In addition to the uplifting influence of parties, there were occasional fun outings. We visited a Japanese garden where we received a guided tour and enjoyed a tea ceremony. Another outing was a city and water tour by amphibious "duck boats," something that none of us had previously experienced although we had known about it for years. On outings, members helped each other by pushing those in wheelchairs or offering carpooling transportation. All of these activities served to make a closely knit, supportive, and caring group.

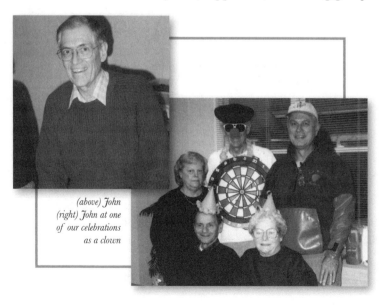

(above) John
(right) John at one
of our celebrations
as a clown

When you have something good going, you want to share it. I invited several friends to attend and observe. My stockbroker brought his wife, a lovely woman in her last stages of cancer. Even without life-limiting illnesses, my daughter, my sister, and even my mother were motivated to attend a Renewal gathering—my enthusiasm was that contagious, I suppose. All were impressed!

I may not have inherited good genes since all four grandparents died of cancer. And none outlived their sixties. Dad dropped dead of a heart attack. But mother was the exception. What should I have learned from her that might extend my own years? For one, she was always open to new information and practices on curing illness and improving the quality of life. That is, she was willing to consider trying something new, if she wanted to do it. That was a factor, I think, in her longevity.

Another was her tough mental attitude. Arriving in America at Ellis Island as an infant immigrant from Western Europe, and without English spoken in the home, she was forced to learn, and to carry her share of family responsibility. Doing an adult's work in a canning factory as a young teenager is probably something now outlawed by work regulations. It wasn't then. Rather than being detrimental to her future, the experience of hard work, swim or sink, seemed to make her tough and resilient. That and, soon after marriage, being confronted with America's Great Depression as a newlywed were akin to tempering the steel in her. Immigrants either learned how to survive in tough circumstances or they withered. Mother became strong.

If I had anything to learn from my mother's longevity I think it was her attitude, possibly her diet, and almost certainly her daily routine. Mother was not necessarily your lovable and compliant old grandmotherly type. She knew what she wanted, what she didn't want, and she'd let you know without diplomacy which was which. We didn't even try to impose on her something to which she was not 100 percent agreeable. Actually, this attitude seems to conform to what science has found to be true of many of the very old. People who question their doctors and form independent choices—not necessarily those "good" patients nor always-agreeable friends—seem to live longer than the more consistently compliant ones. When mother did have a medical problem she refused to accept that it was merely old age and, therefore, incurable. She was willing to try anything if she believed there was even a remote possibility of a cure.

Mother always ate, and served her family, a variety of vegetables and fruits. But she still also ate meat and potatoes, and even had an occasional beer. However, I think that the one most important attribute was that she walked daily with her walker and exercised from her chair using seated arm movements. She kept a grip strengthener by her chair and used it to stave off arthritis even when she passed one hundred years. Previously, in her neighborhood she was known as the old woman who pushed her walker around the block daily, even when it was raining. I know that arthritic knee pain would be excuse enough for many people to stay put in front of their televisions, but not for mother.

She steadfastly refused to accept a motorized scooter or wheelchair to ease mobility in her retirement home. One day when I checked with her about her exercise program. I told her that I, too, had exercised that same day for about 45 minutes, and had also lifted weights for 20 minutes. She advised, "John, I think you are overdoing it. You'd better slow down." Mother was 101 years young and still telling me what to do.

She kept her mind active through membership and play in three bridge clubs until she ran out of transportation options. Also, she was very social. When she saw that the bachelor gentleman across the street had his drinking buddies over for beer and conversation on his front porch, mother would put two bottles of cold beer in her walker and cross the street to join them – notwithstanding an age difference of about 50 years.

Staying involved mentally and physically was important for her. I believe it is a worthwhile lesson for everyone, those who are healthy and those attempting to recover their health. Useful lessons for wellness abound. It may be prudent to study those who have aged successfully and to incorporate into our lives what seems to work. Mother missed seeing her 102nd birthday by one month.

Inevitably the Renewal group attended the funerals of our comrades. But these were usually a cause for a celebration of life, not a morbid recitation of human frailty. It was an opportunity for us to give witness to their wonderful qualities that we had learned first-hand. You would think that by meeting weekly over a period of months or years that we would have learned everything about our friends during their lifetimes. Not so. At one of the first funerals I attended after joining the group I was pleasantly impressed by the high quality of framed photos decorating the walls of the church. It turned out that our departed friend had himself taken the photos. His family wanted us to learn of his previously unknown artistic talent. Humans are indeed deep, and some quite modest.

Shortly after I started attending Renewal, our meeting site was changed from the hospital to an adjacent in-patient hospice center. Dr. DeShazo had been appointed to be the first hospice medical director there and could offer us a comfortable meeting room, space for our expanding library, and ease of parking. Hospice was a new concept for me and, as it later developed, would make an important contribution to my lifelong learning. When a doctor certifies that if a particular disease follows its normal course, a patient probably has fewer than six months to live, that person may elect to receive hospice care. Therapy at that point is out. What hospice offers, at whatever location a patient is in, is comfort and freedom from pain until death takes place. At these two important measures, hospice staffs are the experts. Medicare, it should be noted, provides a free hospice care benefit.

Having thought at one time that I myself could possibly experience an early death I had become interested in end-of-life issues. Hospice programs always need lots of volunteers for various assignments. Here was an opportunity to stretch my comfort zone and increase my knowledge of death and dying. After all, it is an everyday common occurrence but not intimately familiar to most people. I reasoned that I could learn something that would help prepare me for my own future. What I didn't fully realize at the time was how many hundreds of hospice patients, their families, and their friends I would be helping.

After taking the required training I asked for and received placement as a worker in patients' rooms to talk with and comfort them and their families. It was a hugely satisfying experience, so much so that I continued volunteering for ten years. I also became a bereavement worker for spouses of the recently deceased. Truthfully I can say that when the time comes I will have an easier death because of what I have learned from those wonderful people who permitted me to share their precious last weeks and days. The Renewal group enabled me to extend myself and grow in a way I had not dreamed.

If group support is such a good thing, why was it not initially offered to me at the University hospital cancer center where I received my treatment, I wondered. Armed with a conviction that support groups produce good results, I had the audacity to ask my cancer doctor, "Why don't you have a men's support group here at the University?" "You start one and I'll provide the male patients," was his challenging reply. It was easy to form a start-up body of men eager to learn more of a disease that could take their lives. Soon the meeting room was filled each time and men were competing to tell their stories and to ask questions. Being at various stages of diagnosis and recovery, we were learning from each other, i.e., we were providing support.

After the men's group was up and running I returned to Renewal for my personal support. Renewal was more interesting to me because it was attended by a wider cross section of people, both male and female, it featured lecturers on topics helpful to life in general, and Dr. DeShazo was the facilitator.

Having become less uncomfortable with death, dying, and end of life, I decided to take a step back and begin working with people ailing but who might have some hope of recovery. The long-term care ombudsman program is supported in every state of the USA by the Older Americans Act. Ombudsman is a Swedish word denoting an intermediary for a citizen who has a complaint against the government. Here in America it is a person who advocates for the rights of others against all sorts of grievances. In my case, I was trained to help uncover problems that were not otherwise obvious among residents of nursing homes, assisted living facilities, and adult family homes, i.e., state licensed facilities for long-term care. The residents themselves knew that they had problems but, for one reason or another, had not gotten the facility administrator to address them. Identifying complaints to the proper person and seeking an equitable solution was my job.

Sometimes a big problem could find a happy solution with a small effort. I noticed one nursing home woman resident who was taking all of her meals at her bed. She covered her mouth with her hand when she talked. Her dentures no longer fit her and lay in a bedside drawer. She had been eating only minced and pureed food for five months. Of course, she was depressed because, out of embarrassment for having a hollow mouth, she did not socialize with other residents.

As an ombudsman I tried first to empower her to help herself. She was of a generation that "didn't want to rock the boat" by appealing to the staff for help. Her only family, a daughter, was suffering from cancer and "had problems of her own." I simply brought this problem to the attention of the administrator and asked that an appointment be made with a dentist. The next time I saw the resident she was eating at a table in the dining room, enjoying "real food" and conversing with other residents. Her smile revealed both upper and lower dentures. After that she thanked me profusely every time we met. A small input by me dramatically improved the quality of life for that person. I was there to identify the need that others had overlooked.

Because I thoroughly believe in lifelong learning for myself at every available opportunity, I eventually volunteered in all three types of state licensed facilities. I broadened my ombudsman experience and made life more comfortable for those residents. What I had not anticipated was how much this knowledge, gained by defending others rights, would be useful to my friends and even to my own mother when she had to leave her home and move to an assisted living facility. Mother assumed she had lost all of her rights when she moved and henceforth would have to conform completely to what the facility staff told her to do. I knew that the law still gave her definite rights. I became a better caregiver and son to my mother because of knowledge acquired as an ombudsman.

I was learning to advocate.

Because of my ombudsman experience the state Department of Social and Health Services asked me to become a member of its stakeholder advisory council for assisted living. I accepted. My county area agency on aging asked me to join its advisory council for aging and disability services. I served there for three years and further amplified my learning on aging. These networking opportunities made me aware of other approaches to healthy aging. There was an opportunity to instruct people with chronic diseases on how to help themselves suffer less and enjoy life more. Chronic Diseases Self-Management is a nationwide course. I was trained to teach it in hospitals and senior centers. After all, the act of helping oneself is part of what we had been learning in Renewal.

If only we could motivate behavioral change before people got sick we would really be accomplishing a big task, a kind of preventive medicine. I co-founded Sound Steps, a walking program for sedentary seniors that has since been replicated in several cities in the USA and Canada, often by the parks and recreation departments. It was easy to get sponsors to provide T-shirts, water bottles, pedometers and other motivational items. The seniors love them and walk regularly in groups or singly, sometimes charting their progress in notebooks. A Major League Baseball team invited these walkers to use its field "warning track" for exercise. What a wonderful experience to be on the playing field and view the stands as a pro would.

We reasoned that seniors have the time to listen to the radio. We produced 30-second sound bites in which I, as the male voice, talked with a senior woman about health issues. Messages on three health themes are aired on commercial radio in my area. Volunteer activities, which focused on senior health, were a reason, I think, why I was selected as a delegate to the most recent White House Conference on Aging in Washington, D.C. There I rubbed elbows with, and learned from, similarly interested people from all 50 states.

Having started with Renewal, life-threatening illness, death and dying, I seemed to be working in the opposite direction from aging. That is, I was moving toward helping those at an earlier stage of their illness, or, who had no sickness at all. The next step in that direction was to effect health change through legislation. At this point I'll have to admit, with no pride, that I had never talked to an elected official. Of course, I voted. And, sometimes, I complained or made a request by letter or phone. But, I had never talked to a senator, representative, county or city councilmember face-to-face. My attitude was, "This is out of my comfort zone. Let the people who are comfortable talking to politicians do it."

The big change occurred after I signed on to become an AARP volunteer. I was challenged to speak out on a health issue potentially affecting all Americans. At first it required all of my determination to challenge my senator in front of a crowd to reconsider the position she had taken on particular legislation. Eventually, the fact became clear to me: politics is the name of the game. If you don't speak out, you get what those other closed-mouth citizens get, and later complain about it among themselves. If you want to effect big change, you have to state your case to the people empowered to make big changes.

By now I have spoken personally with all of my elected officials on a city, county, state and federal level. I also use e-mail, mail and the telephone and, even testify before committees to support bills that will give us a healthier community and country. We must add our voices for health care for all before we suffer a greater national health crisis. Recognizing my willingness to advocate for quality, affordable health care as well as lifelong financial security, the AARP in my state recently appointed me as AARP state president.

This turned out to be quite a responsible and challenging volunteer job. I chair an executive council that formulates the state action plan for AARP. I am the lead volunteer spokesman for over 930,000 AARP state members. When the legislature is in session I advocate for important senior issues at the capital offices of senators and representatives. I visit congressmen and women to inform them of AARP initiatives and seek their support. I believe that I am using my retirement time to influence for good. All of these health-centered activities had their basis in my experience as a regular attendee and learner at the Renewal meetings.

I have heard survivors say that cancer had contributed positively to their lives. You've heard it said that you have to fall before you can get up again. I can attest that after you have survived a close call, you will carefully reexamine your life. What changes should I make in my daily practices to ensure I will be around a little longer? "You are what you eat" is a saying coined by an early dietician. I considered and modified my food intake. Much good nutritional information was learned at Renewal sessions.

For exercise I now start everyday with 45 minutes of aerobics and stretching. Three days per week I lift weights. I get pneumonia and flu shots and regularly receive medical checks for the common killers of heart, stroke and cancer. A short meditation or nap is a daily practice. I figure that over the years I have invested a lot of time, effort and money in my body. These preventive measures are protecting my investment. Some people, on the other hand, seem to be more occupied with keeping their cars in good shape than their bodies and minds. Let's get our priorities straight!

Hundreds of people who visited Renewal at first scared and suffering or even dying, benefited over the years from the support it provided. And many continued to attend weekly reunions even after the reasons for their original visits had disappeared. They were cured and still coming. Why was this such a magnetic experience? For one, first time visitors were warmly welcomed. Dr. DeShazo always asked them to introduce themselves. He offered them the option of being first of the day to state the reasons for their visit, or to wait until they had observed a few minutes of the reunion and become comfortable.

It was not unusual to devote 20 minutes to a first-time visitor. More seasoned participants would join in to ask helpful questions of newcomers or to offer insights from their own experiences. It is comforting for one just diagnosed, for example, with breast cancer, to be able to talk with someone else who has been there, done that and is still in this world.

For someone suffering, being made the focus of attention by people who really listened and seemed interested was a big draw of Renewal. An even more important factor was that the meeting was led every Monday by an experienced surgeon, Dr. Claude DeShazo. He always reminded that in offering any advice he was not privy to individuals' medical files. However, for me, having him there was like being able to get a second opinion without making an appointment. Or, at the least, it was a seasoned judgment on the course of the chosen therapy. Sometimes he suggested questions that the Renewal participant could ask his or her personal physician.

Upon returning from a professional association meeting, Dr. DeShazo would convey to us the important and useful elements of what he had learned, perhaps a new therapy or a suggestion for disease prevention. Previously I had never been this close up and personal with a medical doctor. Also, he had gotten to know me outside of any consultation room and far more comprehensively than any doctor I could see only in a medical setting. I felt myself blessed by this relationship and better able to control my current and future health. I believe that others had the same feelings.

Renewal had been aptly named. It is true that most of the support group attendees were there as victims of cancer. But some had other diseases, usually life-limiting. Whether they died within weeks or are still surviving and are now healthy, quality was added to their lives by Renewal. Some without disease came simply to become better-informed caregivers for their stricken family members and for their own emotional support. Not every patient is comfortable bringing up his or her personal condition in a group. This is especially true of males.

Health care providers from other facilities sometimes came to observe this successful support group and to build similar groups elsewhere. A man in his 30s and with no apparent health problem attended from time to time. He said that he was unemployed and looking for work. Attending Renewal and witnessing the warmth and support from it, he said, always made him feel better afterwards.

Finally, it has to be said that the founder, Dr. DeShazo is an extraordinary person. Do you know of other doctors who would devote 90 minutes every Monday of the year to meet with people in physical and mental distress who were not their patients? I do not. He started Renewal because he believed that patients had something of value to contribute to other patients over and above what physicians can normally provide. He kept Renewal open and welcoming for many years. We stopped the weekly meetings only after other support groups had been formed in sufficient numbers to accommodate the support needs for the people of the wider community. We still have Renewal reunions whenever we can.

John Barnett is a cancer survivor, recipient of various awards for volunteer work, and author of How to Feel Good as You Age; a Voice of Experience, *published by VanderWyk and Burnham.*

Renewal

CHAPTER 5

THE THINGS THAT
MAKE A DIFFERENCE

"Life can only be understood backwards,
but it must be lived forwards."
— Søren Kierkegaard

We have introduced a number of our Renewal members and talked about some of the meetings. Now let's see if we can state clearly the things that caused our group to be successful. As an introduction, here's part of the letter written to me by Pam H., one of the artists in Renewal, mentioned with her story in Chapter 2. She had both breast cancer and melanoma. Her letter covered her personal story, but additionally was about Renewal and two other support groups where she was actively involved. Some of the letter I have omitted here; this restatement serves as a summary about support groups from one experienced viewpoint. You'll get the idea. Benefits of a support group as seen by Pam H.:

1. Seeing you are not alone in your fear, anxiety, frustration, dread—or in your physical reactions to treatment.

2. Seeing the range of reactions to cancer and to treatment helps to open your eyes to other possible ways to look at your illness and your treatment.

3. Seeing other survivors and patients who are in more serious, dire situations than your own allows more perspective on your own condition... allows you to feel relief and gladness that you're in your situation, not theirs. That's a somewhat mean thought perhaps, but natural.... THESE ARE SPUNKY, ALIVE PEOPLE. They are not numb. They

are inspiring. Life is fragile and uncertain for every one. We cancer patients/survivors are just more aware of it.

4. Good ideas of new areas to explore come from hearing what other participants have found. The attitude of not condemning any idea as quackery, or unlikely to be of benefit, is helpful to me. Who is to say that something is worthless? I'd read books and started my meditation practice, but I didn't know how to judge essiac tea, vitamins, diet, CoQ 10, or herbs. A man I know called me to say he made a device to cure Lyme disease with electromagnetic waves and [in doing so incidentally] had cured an advanced breast cancer! One case of breast cancer! Well, I've learned to go with what makes sense to me and what feels right to me. I've learned to trust my intuition about this medical area. I've learned to rely more on myself to make health decisions. I've read lots of medical books. I have a much more independent ability to judge all treatments. Hindsight being 20-20 I wish I'd never taken hormone replacement therapy for what may have been pre-menopausal insomnia. I'm a much more aware and cautious medical consumer now.

5. I think having a doctor present at the [Renewal] meetings helps keep the group grounded and not off on outrageous stories of miracle cures. The focus is on living well now—learning now.

6. Many people are afraid of death. I have always been afraid of it. We try to ignore it. Since I came to have cancer I've relaxed a great deal about death. I certainly don't want it anytime soon. I'd happily live into my 90s and still be making art. That's my goal. But I do see death as yet another experience. I'm not so terrified anymore—and I don't need to avoid thinking about it. Until then I plan to do a lot of living, doing what I enjoy and what seems meaningful to me. I am a great deal less driven by what other people want of me. I think talking to other people who are facing life-threatening illness and hearing their feelings has contributed to my new attitude.

That is a good summary, but let's drill deeper. We cannot learn everything about everything, but once we identify what is important to us, such as regaining our health, we can look more closely at what will help us. What are the things that make a difference in Renewal?

Voluntary association. Everyone makes their own decision to come to Renewal. In that respect Renewal is like audiences who attend workshops and programs such as the ones featuring well-known authors mentioned in Chapter 8. Nothing will meet everyone's needs, but our group was there on a sustained weekly basis. Many seminars provide excellent material and insight but are soon gone. What was said begins to fade. Over time situations can change too. Members of Renewal knew they could come back and get into discussions about any new development. Everyone felt disease had thrust them into a situation not of their choosing. Members' responses ranged all the way from repugnance concerning the whole situation to a focused desire to learn more. Most members came to supplement conventional treatment with their own efforts. Even the occasional person who took the option of no conventional treatment was moving along with a heavy burden and needed to talk. Our conversations often revealed doubt, second guessing, and recriminations. In difficult moments such as these it helped that members knew everyone in the room was there voluntarily. Members knew they could discontinue coming anytime they chose. And, admittance was free. The only charge was commitment of time and participation.

Renewal was a peer group. As earlier chapters show, we had a wide assortment of members. There were socialites and housewives, professional musicians and manual laborers, newspaper editors, successful business owners and people who had a hard time telling us a single thing they had ever accomplished. We had quite a number of nurses and an occasional physician. They were all peers in either dealing with cancer or being a support person for someone who had cancer. Cancer and a few other chronic diseases were the common denominator in our equation.

Meeting place is not always an option but needs to be considered. Ours was important enough to merit its description at the beginning of Chapter 1. As described in various places, Renewal began by using my office waiting room, then a hospital conference room, then a cafeteria to hold our meetings. All of these places had a different feeling. They sent a message to attendees that our being there was provisional. It was like being transients. This was not intended but may have prompted some urgency by suggesting our meetings might not go on forever. Get what you can while you can.

I was reminded weekly how vulnerable many people feel when they are contending with cancer. In most cases people came into meetings, and not just the initial visit, feeling they did not know anyone. Like most of us do in new situations, our new members looked for cues about how to act. They wanted to find their proper place in a new hierarchy. Until they did, their participation was impeded.

We finally evolved to having a peaceful place where we controlled the immediate surroundings. It offered privacy. We came into a much better circumstance suggesting permanence and could offer a friendly welcome, safety, and a sense of equality. Most of our members had homes and lived conventional lives, but we had a few off the streets or living a very meager existence. The latter especially needed support to begin a new journey.

The quiet of our meeting room was rarely interrupted by anything on the outside or any intrusion. People felt they could get up for a cup of tea or a Kleenex if they needed to. They could linger after meetings and have a private exchange or ask a question. Anyone who might have felt self-conscious in some party garb for our celebrations, or in participating in one of our ceremonies or rituals, did not feel exposed to outside eyes.

We had a permanent place to display our library books and tapes. It encouraged browsing and exploration. Storage capacity made it easy to bring out our pictures of members and events. We could set up quickly for meals or other festive occasions. The privacy of our space, and the sum of all these other things, allowed members to reveal their personal anguish when necessary. So I would say, a meeting space is inanimate but the right place can extend a comforting welcome and allow people a place to breathe.

Self-expression was key to our success. Some people started talking from the moment they sat down at their first meeting. Others took weeks to tell their story or even speak. We all know how difficult public speaking is for most people. Renewal created an atmosphere of safety where even the most reticent individual eventually spoke. LILLIAN was a woman who came for years but never became comfortable in talking. She was very shy. Unfortunately her husband did not care about her problems and somehow Lillian could not get over the feeling she had caused her cancer. She was apologetic and her view of self bordered on shame when she talked about her illness. Still, she would participate. Gradually she became comfortable and when there was a little humor, Lillian would smile and sometimes laugh. She was a very caring woman. Sometimes an "Oh!" would escape her lips when she heard a particularly difficult revelation being voiced in someone else's report. Lillian decided on her own to take the training to become a hospice volunteer. She did that work for a number of years and made significant contributions to others.

Renewal is not about the cathartic release common in the Human Potential movement and similar intense activities. We were not on any clock to get results before time ran out in a scripted weekend agenda. We had time. There was always next week and the next meeting. We were more about clearing away what obscured an individual's true thoughts. We were patiently cleaning dust and grime off a mirror of self-recognition so a member might see themselves. Once that was done we helped that person see the path to what they wanted to become.

Someone once expressed the idea that if the cause of cancer had to be distilled to a single word, that word would be Repression. Whether that is accurate or not, it follows that the antidote for repression should be Expression—expression of self as fully as possible. The Renewal way might take a while, but I believe our way of letting new beliefs supplant old ones one by one was as effective.

Feedback was important to our dynamic. It came from peers; it came in a caring way and in an atmosphere of safety. Most feedback came in terms of someone speaking from personal experiences, or at least having some commonality such as sharing the same diagnosis. It was very powerful when a newcomer perceived that one or more people in the room already had dealt with your own disease or treatment and had something to tell you. Often that newcomer had been attracted to Renewal because they did not know anyone who shared their problems. Such a person thought they were facing the challenge of illness alone.

Our **celebrations** grew in importance over time. They came about in a way that neither I nor anyone else had predicted. The idea started modestly, then expanded to include all the traditional holidays, especially Halloween. Halloween: hide yourself, at the same time, be your self. At their core our parties manifest the natural human desire for merriment. All of us had that desire as children and most lose it as adults. Certainly most people who came to Renewal arrived in the mindset that there was only drudgery ahead. To put on a Halloween costume, or to be planning for days what outfit to wear for the Fourth of July, allowed most members to suspend even legitimate worries. Such celebrations gave credence to principles we discussed like planning an element of pleasure in every single day.

Levity or some pleasurable act needs to be a priority. Humor helps balance our emotions so we can process information needed for survival. Many members reported that they adopted this as part of a new lifestyle. Our celebrations included a potluck meal. Lesser holidays we celebrated with the meal alone. The healing power of laughter and play was put forth in a number of renditions in the 1980s. It was popularized in numerous publications and seminars featuring well-known celebrities. Renewal developed its own adaptation of the theme. Another thing we celebrated was birthdays. There were so many this was done on a collective, monthly basis rather than each week to keep it manageable. Still, it was heartening to see how people lit up when receiving a card, cake with candles, and a moment's recognition.

Ceremony and ritual became as important as anything we did. Much of this had its basis in Native American tradition or lore, but not all. The important thing that happened was our members had these occasions to help them reflect in a different way about self and personal relationships. Some events like lighting candles and remembrances were a way to honor members who had died or had provided inspiration by their personal example. We had the talking stick, the gourd container for holding our annual contracts we made with the future and our candle lighting. We had various totems and relics received from members and healers who visited with us. These ceremonies stopped short of any expiation in a religious sense but they did allow permission to think about future goals and reflect on the past. We had speakers who were healers and ministers. Their various traditions and totems could be powerful tools for stimulating the aspirations of our members.

Forgiveness is such a central concept it needs its own heading. Earlier I identified forgiveness as the key, the key to the lock on our personal door. This psychological door blocks us from getting out and starting our journey to recovery. A central message of Renewal was, begin again from wherever I am. Move forward to be healed. Our healing is not synonymous with the word cure. Cure from our disease is what we commonly say we want. We may not have the faculties to obtain what we want. Healing is a more abstract and multifaceted concept. It may appear as only a substitute objective, and in one sense it is. At the same time healing is broader in scope. It has the potential to take us beyond what we even know now as our goal. Healing is almost always available to us through personal effort. So, let my goal be to heal my self. Let me be renewed. And as a practical reminder,

Those who do not grieve now, grieve later.

All of us have accumulated so much damage and disappointment in living that we are weighed down. Like adding stones to a backpack we proceed through life's experiences adding more troubles. We recall bad things, along with the people and events we blame for causing what happened to us. Unless this pain is examined and processed, lack of resolution keeps our inner door shut. It impedes the process we must begin.

In Renewal the act of forgiveness was a major part of our work. We made it comparatively easy. Once a person's conversations moved to what happened and what went wrong, we could identify the lessons learned. We start along the path, doing the serious work of forgiveness, and the trail takes us to the tree of understanding where we can gather its fruit. Symbolic gestures, rituals and our processes are an adjunct in our renewal work. This is not easy. It is even more difficult because much of it takes place inside us. Personal growth is not a spectator sport.

Surrender. This obscure paragraph may be the hardest to write of anything in this book. Surrender as a concept becomes easier when viewed as part of a continuum with self-awakening, commitment, forgiveness, surrender, then action. Renewal becomes the product. Surrender is difficult to write about because it sounds like giving up, the antithesis of what a cancer patient needs to do. It is not what this book is about. No, surrender in our sense is an actionable step that follows when you do your best and stop worrying about the outcome. This book deliberately mixes stories of successes with what you probably call failures. This is especially true around the issues of disease recurrence or developing a new cancer.

Surrender is leaning into the truth to make our renewal authentic. As I review some of these stories I see instances where people went beyond what you might reasonably think they can do. Some people were intrepid, almost all I consider courageous. Some by comparison seem only to be determined. This process of working on the self was what Renewal facilitated. It was for the kind of people Dr. Bernie Siegel calls exceptional cancer patients. We had a subset of members who could not do for themselves what was necessary and they left. There was a larger group who came to our meetings, got what they needed, then moved on, able now to fend for themselves. Some of the ones we know best were individuals who came for extended periods, years, because they enjoyed interaction with others like themselves. They felt they had something to contribute in an ongoing basis. Surrender in a difficult period of life is equivalent to a second key to our locked door. There is one kind of acceptance required at the beginning, acceptance of what is. Another acceptance, or surrender, comes after you have chosen your new path. It comes when you have done everything possible to make your life successful.

Education and educational materials fill an intellectual need. It gave a quasi-medical legitimacy to what we do in studying cancer as a disease. Discussion of conventional cancer treatment is a practical and legitimate subject. I thought at the outset that such an educational process for our meetings would be the central purpose. As I already have admitted, I was wrong. Learning about cancer certainly is complex enough as a subject. There is science and fact and all the accompanying inconsistencies and arguments about treatment that follow with it. Renewal studied and discussed and tried to stay current. Education went much deeper for all of us than just facts about illness and treatment. There was an elusive truth in our discussions, most of the time flitting just beyond our grasp. Perhaps in our efforts it is best explained in the statement,

Knowing is to becoming as information is to transformation.

Our education and the knowing that came with it we could discuss, dispense, and be conscious of. Transformation and becoming are subtle and often delayed in making their appearance. We need to select from new information things that will help us be a new person. Be eclectic. Your guide probably will be more primitive instinct than intellect. Use your experiences to guide you.

Since so many cancers are preventable, we contended with the issue that developing cancer really is not the patient's fault in the usual sense. The conundrum is, if having cancer is not my fault, maybe I can't fix it. The way out of this is having the courage to take responsibility for doing what we are able to do. Educating ourselves about our disease, investigating what the treatment options are, taking appropriate action, become straightforward educational processes. Looking at what more we can do for ourselves, learning about prevention, going beyond conventional treatment, then sharing what we learn with others, are growth steps. They move us along on our path.

We have already mentioned some of our tools of education. In addition to the lending library and our guest speakers, forums on special subjects added both focus and depth. Less common tools were doing drawings, drawing with the non-dominant hand, the use of body energy, body work, and laying on of hands. There was movement in Tai chi, yoga, and free-form dancing as self-healing art. Among others, Dr. Maria McKinney, who had started the local Music Therapy Center, educated us about specific musical attunements to aid in healing. She shared with us a book she had written, *The Healing Tones of Music*. There is now an extensive bibliography on this subject.

Diet, Exercise, and Meditation are mentioned here because they certainly are important to Renewal. Depending on the individual, any one of these three could be a start on the healing path. These three certainly kept our meeting grounded in practicality. Today so much is written about each of them it is hard to recall how hard it once was to get good information. I still have a list of the books on these subjects I shared with people in the 1970s and 1980s. Diet in overweight America today is approached with optimism about the Sisyphean task of shedding pounds. In Renewal diet centered much more on providing clean-burning fuel for energy or how esoteric molecules in what we ingest serve as catalysts for repair.

Meditation meets with broader acceptability when discussed as stress reduction. Even when we intellectually accept the concept all of us are reticent about change. Such resistance uses energy. We can exhaust ourselves if we do not understand correctly how to change. Quiet times and reflection allow us to recharge. For many of our members this subject involved relearning some convention of prayer used in their youth. For others it was accepting religion for the first time. In the duress of illness, prayer is a conventional way to begin seeking help. Maybe it will help in differentiating these two terms to think of prayer as talking to God and making requests. You have something to say. Meditation is the same physical surroundings but in meditation you remain silent and listen. Meditation creates an open space where God may enter and speak to you.

All three of these, diet, exercise, and meditation, are covered again in the final chapter with some suggestions, so let's leave this subject for now.

Work. Pure and simple, for some people a desire to return to work is the driving force in overcoming illness. In America, someone has observed, work has become the cathedral of our time. If what we value is shown by how we spend our time, then for many Americans our work is what we worship. As a modality aiding healing, it is healthy enough as a goal and conventional enough for our discussions generally to support it.

Recurrence of cancer is another thing that makes a difference in Renewal. From what I have seen, recurrence is the most dreaded aspect of cancer patients' experiences. If this were a game of blackjack, it would be the double down of, "Where did I go wrong?" It highlights the fear we may lose all over again. For some fear of recurrence is the cloud that never goes away. It is the doppelganger accompanying every twinge and ache. It attends follow-up doctor visits and awaits results of routine surveillance testing. Recurrence reminds us of all the emotion attached to the initial illness. That emotion can block our rational consideration of what to do in this new situation. This cannot be dismissed or minimized.

What I can say is, in Renewal, and any other group that creates an atmosphere where challenge is accepted as ongoing, recurrence or a second cancer needs to be put in perspective. Several stories in Chapter 2 were chosen purposefully to dispel the idea that Renewal was some sort of cure-all or had a magic formula. It is true that many people with comparatively straightforward problems and needs came for a time, got what they wanted, then stopped attending. Most of the stories in Chapter 2 are about people with a composite of issues like multiple diseases or the one dreaded the most, recurrence of cancer. It's like all the anguish and effort to this point count for nothing. Suddenly I am reminded I am much closer to the precipice of failure. Call that failure if you want. I believe it is more accurate to say problems arising again or persisting are part of the continuing challenge of life. It was up to our group to understand our selves and our medical system, and the shortcomings of both, as fully as possible.

One of the most influential books ever published in the United States was Viktor Frankl's *Man's Search For Meaning* (1946). Dr. Frankl recorded his memories of the horror and degradation of Nazi concentration camps in WWII. He concluded that no matter how bad things become we make a choice how we will live. He wrote, "...everything can be taken away from a man but one thing: the last of the human freedoms—to choose one's attitude...to choose one's own way." In another place he makes a statement quite apt for us, "When we are no longer able to change a situation—just think of an incurable disease such as inoperable cancer—we are challenged to change ourselves."

People came to us looking for something. This was true even when they didn't know what that something was. This book is more about self-realization, self-assessment, and self-reliance than an intricate dissection of cancer as a disease process. It also is not a specific formula for cure. It is a chance to make the person, not the disease and not the physician, the most important thing. Every Renewal member had some association with physicians. Many of these relationships continued throughout the experience. Outside our meetings most members would agree, existence is a dynamic triangle between the disease(s), the physicians, and one's own personal interests. The point of focus and width or scope of the triangle's angles vary over time.

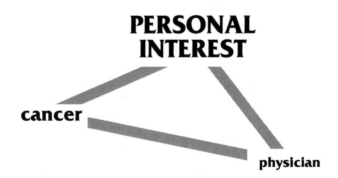

PERSONAL INTEREST

cancer

physician

Our personal interest is larger than our disease. It is the most important thing. The physician is an adjunct and our advisor. He or she has a more limited scope of interest, does not have the perspective to see everything, and is not the one to be in control. Cancer is one-dimensional, weak, and interested only in self-propagation.

This book presents various ways to explore and learn more. We do not have to overlay Renewal in this diagram in an egocentric way. It is enough to suggest that seeing a person's goals, their very being, as separate from both the disease and the physician is the important thing. Disease and suffering are not things we consciously choose. They insinuate themselves into our lives by a combination of environmental factors, habits, and hereditary predispositions. Disease exists in a self-centered way. Cancer certainly is not the conscious culmination of what we want for a future. Disease becomes our opportunity for self-examination: "What is the lesson here?" If there is a recurrence or new illness the question becomes, "What lesson have I not learned yet?"

Hospice might legitimately be omitted from this list but for our group it was part of our educational process. I got involved in founding a hospice in our community after Renewal started. When built it was an attractive facility offering privacy, pleasant surroundings, and lack of a hospital's usual clinical goals. For more than a decade it is where we met. The very meeting portrayed in Chapter 1 took place in our hospice setting. Several individuals presented in chapters that follow were involved in hospice but bridged across to their other work in nursing, oncology, and psychiatry.

For people who came to Renewal hospice was an introduction to a novel concept. Here is exposure to the final step in a person's life. Due to its proximity members could explore in their own time or ignore it. Being in the same physical setting where hospice care was carried out provided a gentle reminder of another difficult subject: we are all going to die. It is possible to separate death from experiencing cancer—just keep focusing on getting well. For many in Renewal dealing with disease itself was an eye-opening occurrence. As part of its instructional value, cancer leads to deeper reflection upon how this will end up for all of us.

Some of our members wound up in hospice care. Most who do so stay at home and never enter a dedicated facility such as ours. The other part of this exposure to hospice was showing people that their second great fear after recurrence, pain and/or loss of control in life, were things that can be managed successfully.

Renewal

CHAPTER 6

BENDING THE BRANCH

"Go confidently in the direction of your dreams!
Live the life you've imagined. As you simplify your life,
the laws of the universe will be simpler."
— *Henry David Thoreau*

The next three chapters deal in various ways with physicians and other caregivers. Before getting into some of that I want to share with you several of my formative experiences, things that changed my attitude as a practioner. This is scaled back from any detailed experience of being a practicing surgeon. Books by surgeons and other physicians about their training and their practice are commonplace, as are recommendations about health issues. My purpose is to sharpen your perception about physicians and make your decisions about them more conscious.

What follows is meant to help you better understand your personal caregiver as a person. This theme continues through additional perspectives in Chapters 8 and 9. I want to get you re-thinking your experiences and considering new avenues for reaching health goals. Use this chapter as an aid in reflecting upon formative events in your own life, illness, and people who are treating you. Doing so may help you understand who you have become. Such thinking in the presence of current adversity may give both new direction and options for your own path toward renewal. My intention is to turn whatever is before you now into something positive, something worthwhile and rewarding.

A metaphor flashed in my mind just as I began writing this chapter, how impressionable I was in my early medical career. Events recorded here changed what happened in my later life. Similarly, early bending of branches on a tree can alter its mature appearance markedly. With such thoughts in mind I decided to use this comparison and call this chapter about myself Bending the Branch.

This sequence in thinking probably arose because in 1987 I took up bonsai work as an avocation. I liked it. Then in 1995 I bought a farm and started growing apples commercially. I studied intensive orcharding and the use of espalier techniques for directing growth. I had over 3000 trees I was continually training. The orchard became an opportunity to shape growth on a much larger scale than the bonsai work. It was peaceful, away from my busy other life. Orchard work had kinesthetic qualities and taught me skills for shaping growing things. Like any garden, growing apples offered an orderliness of mind, esthetics, and had utilitarian value.

On the professional side I can look back now on my exuberance in becoming a physician. It was all I ever wanted to do. Two decades later I started Renewal. Now even that is almost 30 years past. Forty-five years after becoming a physician I am turning back to events that may help you understand the concept of renewal in a different way.

Your experiences are different from mine, of course, but all along they have been shaping you. I hope what follows will bring you to a new self-examination.

I'll begin with two out-of-the-ordinary things that happened to me in medical school. The first was being put in a very unusual relationship with the chairman of our Department of Medicine. This man carried the dual titles of Department Chairman and Physician-in-Chief for the medical center. Most of the time he was referred to simply as "The Chief."

Nothing was as stressful as making clinical rounds with The Chief and being vulnerable to an ambush of sudden questioning. He had a knack for sensing a hapless student's lack of knowledge about some esoteric point—he read it in our eyes—then exposed it. His learning and experience were vast, ours just beginning and unsure. These were encounters that could escalate to confrontations with our ignorance. They led to mumbling, downcast eyes, and sweat-provoking exchanges for me. At best they led to embarrassment watching a classmate being intellectually peeled like a banana. The Chief was tall and severe in his appearance which added to his intimidation factor. He was never seen revealing a conventional smile.

When a moment of humor required response, The Chief's lower jaw dropped slightly, exposing his lower teeth in an expressionless way and a monotone "Ha, Ha, Ha" rolled out.

These teaching rituals turned to academic turmoil in the summer before our third year. The Chief was diagnosed with bone cancer. It was an osteosarcoma in his right hip. He was whisked away to a specialty hospital in New York City for definitive surgery. In order to remove the tumor not only half of the pelvic bone but also his thigh and lower leg had to be sacrificed. Back at the medical school we got periodic reports forecasting an early return to his clinical duties, but shortly after The Chief returned home, follow-up x-rays showed a metastasis had already appeared in one lung. Statements followed saying removal of the lung tumor would soon take place. This news made its way furtively down to us plebeians like medical gossip. It became the central topic of discussion in the hospital and entire medical community.

Before resection of the lung metastasis could be carried out, neurological signs indicated the fast-growing tumor had spread to his brain. This succession of developments destroyed all prospects of cure. At home The Chief was being cared for by his wife and she was fast becoming exhausted. When word got out how much of a toll all this was taking on his spouse, one of my classmates suggested that several of us third year students take turns staying overnight with The Chief, removing the necessity of hiring nurses. I was one of the ones asked to join the cadre for this duty. The wife insisted upon paying us as if we were nurses, which was welcome income to us impoverished students—it was $25 a night, I believe. But none of us had any idea what we were getting into.

With the wife's help a plan was agreed upon. One of us students was to show up each evening at 7 o'clock and stay until 6 o'clock the next morning. At that point the wife would take over for the day and we could return to the hospital in time for our next day's duties. The couple had no children. The only other resident in their house was The Chief's father, a retired and very elderly homeopathic physician. The Chief, now our patient, had been moved to a separate bedroom so his wife could sleep.

So we started. Our patient was in the spare bedroom. It had only indirect light from the adjoining bathroom. This arrangement was to encourage rest, but it added a continual gloom and incipient depression to the work we were doing. The great learning of this entire experience came from my sitting in this darkened room, essentially having no duty except to be present for the needs of someone else.

We were there to do whatever was necessary to keep the Chief comfortable. We were to avoid letting him become agitated, a problem as pressure from his brain metastases grew and affected his thinking. At unpredictable times this phenomenon appeared like a cloud moving in front of a brilliant intellect, then passed on.

I learned practical things such as how morphine tablets taken for pain caused dry mouth. Every few minutes water had to be provided. "A sip of water," The Chief would say hoarsely, then roll his tongue awkwardly to capture the straw in the glass being offered. This went on all night, interrupted by periods of fitful sleep. There was awkwardness in every act, such as using a urinal or bedpan. I had to support and mostly lift when he insisted on moving to the commode chair. This was doubly difficult since one half of his pelvis had been reduced to little more than a socket. There was no stability and I was panicky about the consequences of a fall.

Then came peaceful interludes when The Chief wanted to discuss medical esoterica or have something read to him. All hope of a successful outcome had disappeared but the existence of The Chief's towering intellect had not. Mostly I just sat quietly at the bedside in the gloom.

The Chief's condition deteriorated. There was no one else to vie for the wife's attention and at irregular intervals she would rise during the night and come to check on her husband. She obviously cared deeply for him. They really only had each other. I often wondered, watching her retrace steps to her bedroom, what must it be like, having the social status conferred on the wife of such a highly regarded man fade away to this?

During these several months before The Chief died of his brain metastases there was one other regular night visitor: his father. The father, as I mentioned, was a retired homeopathic physician. In those early days I didn't even know what a homeopath was. The Chief was this elderly gentleman's only child. The father had decamped and moved to live in his son's house. The anguish he felt over the situation was evident though never articulated. The father became a night wanderer like the wife, appearing at intervals to check on what he now considered his patient too. The father had been relegated to clandestine visits. Differences of opinion between him and the allopathic physicians actually in charge of The Chief's case put him on the outs. The father, clinical philosophies aside, was somewhat befuddled because of age and sorrowful to see his only child slowly dying before him. He was determined to do something. He might be caricatured by the "regular" doctors, but the old man had his beliefs and remedies coming from a very different clinical experience. The father's only opportunity to try his ideas was during the night when there was neither scrutiny by a day nurse nor the wife.

When the father came in with his potions, the old gentleman would try to explain to me what this or that was supposed to do. I was still grappling with conventional pharmacology and didn't grasp what he was trying to accomplish. This did become my first exposure to compromise in medical care based upon differing clinical judgments. I came down on the side of believing the father's nostrums wouldn't hurt. I, and I presumed my fellow students, just stood by in these moments. The elderly physician cajoled his son to take a few sips of this, or put a few drops of that under his tongue. There was a palpable sense from The Chief, when he was lucid, that he didn't believe in all this, but he too submitted to his father's wishes.

I relate such private events now because, almost fifty years after they took place, I am trying to explain myself. I didn't think anyone would be harmed by what I allowed to happen. Because I, as both an impressionable medical student and young man who at the time had no son of my own, came to see the love between father and son as a unique circumstance—even if between them the word love was never spoken.

Another lesson in this early experience of care-giving was the wide swings of emotion that taking care of this once-feared teacher caused within me. If there was one word most of us medical students had to describe our experience of The Chief, that word would be fear. Then, sitting at his bedside in a hard-backed chair, dozing off when I could, there would be tranquil moments when the Chief would awaken and want to talk. Maybe I would read something aloud for a while until he dozed off. Then there were the water sipping rituals. I fretted when he said he wanted another pain pill right now but it was still twenty minutes before time. I would check his record to see if dispensing another pain pill was coming too soon, mindful that a request from him was not really a request but a directive. What if I were to be responsible for an overdose and killed him?

Somehow he and I successfully negotiated about the pain pills. Sometimes I was evasive and tried to change the subject; sometimes I just gave him what he wanted. Even with our unbalanced status I came to realize the powerful thing conferred upon any person assuming a role as caregiver.

When the chief roused himself he might suddenly become alert and businesslike with musings like, what did I think he should do about some administrative decision in his department? Or, he would inject, "I've got to get over this thing." He asked my opinion about if I thought he should have brain radiation, or, what did I think his chances were? Just as quickly he'd lapse again into incoherence. As the pressure inside The Chief's head grew worse, further dimming the thought processes of a brilliant mind, there could be some unpredictable moments like these and I felt a rush of anxiety. I swung from being caregiver in charge, the physician on duty, back to being a know-nothing. I was the student once again, scrambling to avoid academic disaster. I look back now and see the fear existed only within me. I learned a steady hand and a calm voice, when I could muster those, were powerful instruments for establishing roles in difficult situations.

I was very impressionable back then having little frame of reference as to how to act. What the experience did teach me was that all of science will only take you so far. Being human and showing understanding are equally important in being effective.

The second, equally formative thing in medical school happened the following year. As our class finished our third year we moved closer to being baptized legitimate physicians. Eight of us were offered employment at the Mississippi State Hospital at Whitfield. In addition to being paid a handsome $200 for each of the summer months, we were able to continue throughout the senior year on night/weekend call basis and be paid for that too. We eight were essentially being extended an offer to practice medicine. We were under the supervision of the institution's staff but it was a degree of independence roughly on the level of being a resident physician.

In those days people with serious mental illness routinely were committed to Whitfield. For decades state residents associated the name Whitfield with being the state's repository for the mentally ill. It was a huge facility. The hospital provided institutional care for about 5000 patients. It had its own medical and dental staff and functioned like a town of comparable size. It housed patients with every known psychiatric diagnosis and it was fascinating to study them. The inmates ranged from people with congenital defects and metabolic problems like cretinism to depression, senility, and what we probably would diagnose now as Alzheimer's disease. There were all manner of psychoses, schizophrenia and manic states. It housed murderers, rapists, a whole building of criminally insane.

Within this larger institution was a small hospital divided into separate wards for men and women. Here patients with acute medical diseases could be admitted and cared for under the supervision of staff internists and on-call specialists. During the summer months I actually was assigned a small ward of my own. In those days the Physician's Desk Reference was a reliable clinical aid superior to a textbook. It, along with a Merck Manual plus our standard textbooks and making daily rounds with an experienced internist, enabled me to make my own treatment decisions.

After hours and on weekends, one of us would be charged with recording our clinical activities in a log book. We also had a staff car to cover the expansive institutional grounds. Depending upon their diagnosis and/or risk of leaving the grounds, patients lived in open cottages or more secure ward-like buildings. Each building had its own staff nurse and attendant. The criminally insane were locked up just like in prison but otherwise things were pretty open. Once the day staff left it was like being the only doctor for a small town. All of us senior students were mature enough to enjoy being given our first real taste of practicing medicine. It was us versus the challenge of disease. It was a moment having clarity of purpose. The battle was on! I still look back upon that time with fondness.

Of all the hundreds of learning experiences I had at Whitfield that year, the most enduring memory is how I came to appreciate my relationship with the nurses. Whitfield was definitely an unusual situation, but I have never forgotten the human characteristics of nurses there. I came to temper any feeling of clinical autonomy with the realization that practicing medicine is a play with many roles. I learned to value the observation and experience of others. I learned to listen and to value teamwork.

The treatment protocol for acute illness within this mental facility community began with an on-duty registered nurse. Like those of us acting as the doctor on call, the duty nurse had a log book and car and responded to the calls first. I have no idea how many times I got to sleep in the duty quarters while the nurse made a treatment decision and never awakened me. I never challenged this arrangement because I always needed sleep. What I did get to witness was how good these women really were in diagnosis and treatment.

There were several experienced registered nurses doing this work. The ones I remember most are the two who were usually on duty, one or the other, on the nights and weekends I worked. Maybe it was coincidence; maybe they scheduled it that way. The important thing is, I knew when they called me, somebody needed help. Later in my practice I came to realize how many health professionals cannot differentiate between who is sick and who is not—what is important and needs immediate attention and what does not.

I came to call these two women and a few others like them, the "night nurses"—as if working at night itself conferred some special degree of wisdom and practicality. When one of these nurses called all she had to say in verbal shorthand was something like, "You better come over to Cottage ____, or building such-and-such." With that simple phone call I knew to be out the door and on my way. Sometimes in difficult or primitive conditions, like a padded cell where the patient was in the process of shredding the covering off the wall, I wouldn't know what to do. With their working knowledge of almost every one of these 5000 patients, the nurse might give me a gentle hint, prodding me with information like, "He (or she) had a spell like this last week and here's what worked back then..." Or, gave some moderating bit of advice like, "Maybe we should come back and check on him in a couple of hours and see how he's doing." So we might not do anything just when I was about ready to hit the panic button. Patience, the nurses suggested, often allowed the problem to take care of itself.

The nurses addressed me as doctor, something always welcomed by an evolving medical student. They enforced a discipline on the lesser staff making sure they knew that I, the doctor, had said to do something. Those orders were to be followed. Still, if their thirty-plus years of experience in this work told them my decision was off, I knew it in an instant. All it took was the nurse's glance directed my way below slightly raised eyebrows. No one else could see this signal taking place but I knew it was up to me to decide which of us had the better idea.

The next best part of working with these older nurses was the personal relationship we developed. I say older because I was still in my early twenties. Each of them was old enough to be my mother and all of us knew it. I suspect they looked at me like a son, especially the two nurses I mentioned. Sometimes when they both happened to be on duty because of the work load, we would sit down together in the dingy kitchen of some cottage and drink coffee. A steaming pot was always there as the staple offering. It tasted so good after we dealt with some crisis. It might be late at night or early in the morning. We'd still take time to talk, not only about the diagnosis, which medical school convinces you is the paramount issue, but about the person we had just seen and what their personal story was.

Maybe one of the nurses knew that the underlying problem was some family member had visited the problem patient the previous day and gotten him or her riled up. Maybe trouble started with some squabble in the day room over which TV channel to watch. Maybe it was a conflict in personality between the patient and a staff member. What I pondered as a perplexing set of clinical signs or symptoms more often than not had a story behind it and a psychological twist. I looked at the clinical part; these women looked at the whole picture. Gradually they taught me how to do the same.

Night hours, coffee, and cigarettes were our routine. Both these older nurses smoked every chance they got. Ever practical, they smoked Raleigh cigarettes. Back then part of the small talk included what gifts to redeem with coupons that came with each pack. I think there were four extra coupons included if you purchased a carton of cigarettes at a time—as they usually did. At any rate these women found a ready audience in me for all the stories they had to tell. They readily shared their cigarettes with me, the impecunious medical student. Under the glare of a bare light bulb or some humming fluorescent tube, there we would sit, drink coffee and smoke. How I appreciated what those women taught me about practicing medicine! Those nurses taught me more than they ever knew.

After graduation I went to the University of Minnesota Hospitals for a straight surgical internship. I had begun my formal surgical training. Internship today is incorporated as the first year in surgical residency. Back then it was a survey of the various sub-specialties and usually had a rotation through twelve different disciplines. Three things stand out in memory from that year:

My first month was on the urology service. During that first rotation I remember taking a history and doing a physical exam on an attractive girl about 18 or 19 years old. I think she stands out because she was very fit and did not look in the least like she needed to be in a hospital. She had been a high school athlete in several sports she told me. She certainly looked like she was stronger than I was. Some routine blood tests done in her hometown had uncovered something very wrong. She had been referred to the medical center for workup of renal failure. There was no physical evidence of any problem; she was the youngest person I had ever seen with end stage renal disease.

My second month was a ward assignment across the street from the main hospital. That separate building had a cavernous open room with curtain dividers between the beds. It was called a cancer ward, the first time I had ever encountered the term. It was also my first sustained contact with cancer patients. The daily census varied from about 20 to 30 people. In essence this was where all the patients receiving chemotherapy were assigned to be sure they were cared for by the most experienced staff. Interns were the flunkies and did not make important decisions about therapy regimens. We were there for two things. One was to administer chemotherapy cocktails intravenously, making sure none got outside the veins to cause tissue damage. The other duty was, since the medications and all the blood tests soon used up all of a patient's veins, to get creative and be sure there was a vein somewhere to administer the treatments and draw blood samples. For my second month, that person was me.

I don't want to make this sound worse than it was, but this ward was a big room, not air conditioned, and August in Minneapolis is hot. In this big space every sound carried. Whatever happened was shared, even if it did happen behind some privacy curtains. Every wince, every whimper, every groan or plea to negotiate a moment's delay carried. It was shared as part of the ward's collective experience. This was my first encounter with people who acted repulsed by, not thankful for, the treatment they were given. That attitude confused me; it was inconsistent with what I thought I was doing there.

The nurses and other ward staff reported for their duty shift. They came and went. I and others like me got called to make the injections and deal with other problems. There were very few visitors. The ones who did visit seemed unsure of how they were supposed to act. Most appeared uneasy in these surroundings. The senior medical staff, the decision-makers, came by occasionally but their stays were brief. Changes in medication were made but the whole atmosphere was one of a holding pattern, distorted as if there were no end point or goal, as if time didn't matter.

To make so many individual injections was very time consuming. It took half the day. The elapsed time seemed even longer because this was a lonely place. Almost every patient had something they wanted to talk about. Each one had just finished lying in bed for another 24 hours and time revolved around the pain of injections and blood draws. Patients liked talking to me because I was a fresh face. There was little conversation between people in adjacent beds. When patients turned to see who was in the next bed they saw a cancer patient, and it scared them.

A lot of what I did became a negotiation: "I don't feel well; can't we skip today's injection?" someone would ask. "Couldn't you come back a little later?" It affected me that I was the chief cause of their pain; I was the one seen as inflicting it. There were many mundane yet practical things to learn, mostly dealing with constipation, sore mouths (usually a yeast infection), and getting creative with pain medication. I always appreciated after that month what oncologists do. They deal with these issues of pain and disappointment every day.

At the end of my internship year I came off the services doing surgery and had an assigned rotation principally doing wound care. The university hospital was a regional referral center and received many patients with terrible problems. Many of them had extensive surgical procedures. Some operations did not work and fell apart. Those patients got deep abscesses and terrible wound infections and tissue loss. The thinking at the time was that all such infected patients needed to be isolated from the non-infected ones. So anyone with a wound infection got transferred to a new service and then to me. Once again, I had adequate supervision from the residents and staff, but once my superiors saw I was competent, the rest of the service drifted off to other assignments and left the wound infections to me. Somehow I think I had telegraphed that I saw all these open wounds as a challenge.

This too was an open ward. In addition to my rolling table of instruments and supplies I moved an articulated curtain divider around with me from bed to bed. And again, every patient on the ward formed a concept of the intimate details of everyone else from what they could hear spill over the curtains from the beds nearby. I had never seen wounds with pus and necrosis like this before. I started out with some trepidation, but grew more confident with what I was doing with each passing day. It is not an exaggeration to say that there were abdominal wounds extending up under the diaphragm or to the bottom of the pelvis which required me to go up to my elbows in reaching their limits.

There are basic principles of wound care: cut out dead tissue, create adequate drainage of pus, use of antibiotics and change bandages as often as necessary. I devised some novel approaches to wounds. I took pride in how wounds started to heal, but there was no one to share these satisfying moments with except an occasional nurse or orderly. I was free to test some of my theories about using vitamins and the trace element zinc as supplements to aid in patients' recovery. By the end of the second week one patient was well enough to go home. Soon thereafter another one left. By the end of the month every person there on the first day of my rotation had been discharged, though emptied beds had started to fill again.

One who did not make it home was a girl I didn't recognize at first. I knew right away that this was a problem case because the young woman was drawn up in a fetal position. She wailed and pulled back as soon as I or anyone else touched her. She was emaciated but refused to eat. Across her lower abdomen was an open wound from a failed kidney transplant. It took three days of cajoling before I could treat her. Then it hit me: this was the healthy-looking young woman I had done the admission workup on last July. After rotating off that service I had forgotten about her.

It took a while to review the woman's chart at the nurse's station. The old chart had grown to be six inches thick. I looked back to follow the chronicle of how she had lost her transplant after a protracted battle with rejection. She actually had a second kidney transplant and it too had been rejected. Her immune system was devastated and now she had gotten this infection. She was without any kidney function and being maintained on dialysis, something she never experienced prior to entering the hospital.

The young woman clearly didn't remember me either. I was just another white uniform to her now, and she had seen too many of those in all these months. She was my greatest challenge on the ward through that month because she didn't care. "Just leave me alone!" was about all she would say.

I came in one morning and noticed that this woman's bed was empty. "Where is she?" I asked the head nurse.

Apparently the commotion had cleared only shortly before my arrival at 7:00 a.m. The head nurse told me the girl had been discovered lifeless by one of the nurses on early rounds about 6 a.m. In a way we all felt relief that this particular ordeal had ended.

As with any unanticipated death, an autopsy is a matter of standard procedure in a teaching hospital. It was about noon when I got a call from the pathology resident doing the autopsy. He questioned me keenly for a minute or two. I thought his tone of voice was odd. Then, detecting that I was being straightforward and had nothing to reveal, he explained his call. "She died of an air embolus," he told me. "Something didn't look right," he went on before I could think of anything to say, "so I opened her heart under water. It was full of nothing but air." Clearly this was not something which would have happened by itself.

As I hung up the phone I turned, with no particular intent, to announce to the staff what I just had been told. The faces looking at me were impassive. No one said anything. Everyone turned back to their work. I knew something was wrong. Why weren't they eager for the details or showing any reaction? After a moment I realized it was because they already knew.

Later one of the nurses told me. She made an oblique reference suggesting the possibility air had been injected accidentally into the woman's intravenous line sometime during the night. The exact circumstances and who did it, I don't know. Maybe the patient herself implored someone to end her misery. I felt certain it was an act of compassion. This woman was someone who suffered tremendously and had no hope of recovery. What happened was quiet, it was painless, and one life passed on during the night. I never followed up to see how the formal pathology report explained the findings. It was written up I'm sure, but there was no momentum for an investigation. The patient was gone.

I'm going to fast-forward ten years. It was essentially a time of prolonged surgical training with many thousands of experiences. It also includes my two year service in the U.S. Navy with a year in Vietnam with the Marines. More changed in my life during that year with a Marine battalion in combat than in any other time period of my life, but that is not part of the Renewal story.

Toward the end of those ten years I spent one year back at the University of Minnesota training to be an organ transplant specialist. Most of the people we cared for had the hepatitis B virus in their system because of blood transfusion and dialysis. It was endemic, as we say. One minor needle stick when I helped a resident perform an operation resulted in my being inoculated with that pathogen. After several months of incubation my hepatitis became clinically apparent.

At first I did not know what was wrong with me. I had nausea and fever then progressed to severe weakness and lassitude. I developed intense itching and a generalized rash. Then one morning my urine was the color of Coca Cola. Suddenly I knew what was wrong. I could hardly believe it. I was sick with something serious just as I was about to start my first real job as a professor! After that my eyeballs turned yellow and my entire body took on a dingy yellow hue. I saw a local physician who specialized in liver problems and he confirmed my diagnosis. There was nothing he could prescribe; treatment was all a matter of rest and waiting.

I was in bed for several months. I had no appetite and the feeling of weakness was profound. Sunlight was too bright for me to go outside. My eyes ached so much I could neither read nor watch television. My liver grew huge. It had an odd way of rolling back and forth when I turned over. I would get restless in one position and roll to the side. Several seconds later my liver would follow creating a sloshing sensation in my distended belly. It was impossible to eat anything with fat in it. Even the aromatic oils in brewing coffee made me start to heave.

After three months my weakened body recovered enough to get up but it took another year for my liver to recover. I went to a gym and started lifting five pound weights. I had never been so weak. When the liver cannot produce glycogen as an energy reserve exertion causes sudden episodes of profound weakness. When such spells hit me, I had to find a place to sit down fast or I would collapse.

I won't go on about this. For all these years I have felt that such a serious illness helped me to understand when a patient tries to explain a vague but profound loss of energy. Having hepatitis B was a gift. It gave me empathy and at least a visitor's pass to understanding where my cancer patients and Renewal members lived. This brings us up to the mid-1970s. After I left my academic career at the University of Washington I went into private practice in a Seattle suburb.

Part of the reason medicine can be such a wonderful profession, such an adventure, is that every practitioner gets to encounter thousands of individuals as patients. Some people say they want to travel the world to see different sights and meet interesting people. Physicians can get the same thing by just being attentive to daily life when they come to their offices. We get to view our patients' diseases in their infinite variety. If we listen, we also get to hear the story of those peoples' lives. We can learn from the sum of their experiences and that offers a tremendous education. If we are up to it, and open to it, we can meet and interact with whole families. It's the easiest pathway I know on this earth to becoming wise.

One of my surgical mentors told me of his experience years before of keeping a private list of every operation he ever did. "Then one day," he said, "I added the ten thousandth case to my list." He paused for a moment in the telling, "Then I realized that was enough record keeping. It was enough; and I quit."

That statement had special meaning to me because up to then I was doing the same thing. I had begun a record of every case dating back to the first operations I was allowed to do at Whitfield hospital and during my internship. I was in private practice when my older friend recounted this story from his past. By coincidence it was the exact time I had added number ten thousand to my own personal list. He could not have known about my record keeping but this man, Dr. Jim Gallant, was the wisest surgeon I ever knew. I heard this story from his experience and I got it. I was just keeping a list and making it longer. It was an ego thing and accomplished nothing. So I stopped.

In private practice I was developing a local reputation for being somebody who was good. Trouble was, I had become too successful too fast. The first six months after I opened my practice I made rounds in the hospital twice a day, seven days a week, and never took a day off. I operated all the time, had over twenty patients in the hospital most of the time, and making rounds alone took hours. Those were the times that people stayed in the hospital for a week after gallbladder removal and several days after hernia repair.

I kept getting busier and busier. General surgeons as a group have a hard time saying "No" to any referral or opportunity that comes their way. Back in those days a surgeon had some control over what he or she got paid, so you could also make a good living while doing what you liked to do. There was always time to add one more case. So I kept doing more and more, crowding in extra appointments over lunch and at the end of the day. I started having office hours on Saturday, trying to always be available. Part of what saved me was taking in several partners to spread the volume of work, but then we were always assisting one another, so the net time spent working never decreased.

For a time I prided myself on how efficient I had become. I could take a phone call from a referring doctor between two exam room visits almost without breaking stride. In the hospital I could hold a phone to each ear, keeping two conversations going by swinging first one receiver, then the other, down to speak. I streamlined my approaches to patients, but some things just couldn't be hurried. Talking about a hernia repair could be rote when you have done it 500 times, but for the patient it was the first time. When a patient was trying to understand about having their colon removed, well, what does that mean? Does it mean I have to wear a bag? And no matter how carefully a surgeon enters a conversation about breast biopsy, the very mention of breast surgery releases a flood of apprehension to many women. A lump, a spot, a lesion, whatever you are calling it, could it be…cancer? These were things people wanted to know. I had created a busy and successful world. I kept thinking about how much I had to hurry. Many opportunities for relationships were being lost.

I was doing a lot of complicated cancer and vascular cases—more than most surgeons would predict for a community hospital. It was as if our clinic had become a referral center on its own. The concept of a teachable moment certainly did not originate with me, but I came to recognize it and appreciate what it was. There just wasn't enough time for me to listen to all that patients wanted to say. So I started keeping my little library of educational and self-help books I mentioned before. Feedback convinced me this drawing closer to patient needs had relevance. Some things patients wanted to know more about, I just needed to find a way to let them hear.

What had begun to change in me was made possible by my staff. I found teachable moments with inquisitive patients whenever I looked. Instead of parsing things and saying, "Come back and see me in two weeks," I started staying until all a patient's questions were answered. When the usual visit time was up, or my nurse knew in advance of a patient's concern, she would put her ear near the door to judge by the tone of the voices inside whether a serious conversation was underway. At first my running over 15 minutes, 30 minutes, or more, caused inconvenience with our scheduling. In such instances the nurses knew to tell the receptionists to start making adjust-ments—I was at it again. Bless them. Just as nurses in the hospital looked out for both my patients and me, the women in my office took care of me too. First there was Lynn, then Helen, then Rebecca, Nancy, and Linda. Out front there was Rachael, our receptionist, and Teri, my office manager. All of them kept some semblance of order and decorum and yet made it pos-sible for me to stay focused on what I wanted to do. Bless them all.

The magic of this was, most of the time, patients understood. Not everyone, of course. Some people got mad if they had to wait. They acted out or threatened to leave before being seen. But most seemed to know that even with a delay, their time would come. They would get their turn. They came to know we were not going to close and go home until everyone was seen. Over time the nurses became so expert that if I were called away for an emergency they met with patients and fielded phone calls on their own. Their answers and reassurance alone satisfied many patients. Sometimes it was just a matter of taking a look at an incision and doing a bandage change, or taking out sutures when it was time. Lynn and Helen especially had the knack of seeing people on their own. They often made unsolicited calls to patients to inquire as to how they were doing. These nurses were so good that many patients would see them and be satisfied without seeing me at all.

I kept probing for ways to make patients understand the ramifications of whatever disease they had. It was education and also an exploration of new possibilities. Forget about blame and whose fault this is. Forgive everyone you know. Move on. Do something for your self. More challenging was trying to explain what might be an opportunity hidden in this disorder—even if its name is cancer.

One thing I tried for a while was posting a placard over the exit door. It said, "DON'T LEAVE THIS OFFICE UNTIL ALL YOUR QUESTIONS ARE ANSWERED." It was intended to give people permission to stop, come back, to make the most out of every office visit.

For a while I started giving health-related lectures to the public. Even when I felt I did a good job, it felt like preaching. Like most sermons I have heard in my life, even the best make a temporary impression, then are blurred by the activity of life and soon forgotten. Years later I read an editorial by the newly-named editor of *Time* magazine as he introduced himself to his readers. I have forgotten his name, but feel he got the sentiment just right. He prefaced his point of view about guiding his publication by saying he had grown up in New Orleans. Southern men he went on to say, when they get to be a certain age, mature into one of two things. They either become preachers or they become storytellers. Based upon results up to that time I knew I didn't want to become a preacher about health. So I needed to find some way to take the wealth of stories about patient lives and activities and keep it from being lost. Right now you are holding my best effort in doing that.

Another thing I did was change my professional business card. I got the idea from a physician in Chicago whose name I have since forgotten. What he told me about in Chicago traveled with me to Seattle. He encouraged me to copy what he did. So, on the back of my business cards, instead of lines to write the next appointment, a revised printing gave these seven bits of advice:

- RESPECT YOUR BODY
- TAKE TIME TO RELAX
- ACCEPT YOURSELF
- SHARE YOUR TRUE SELF
- CREATE LIFE GOALS
- LOVE UNCONDITIONALLY
- BE SPIRITUAL

Recently I visited with a doctor friend still practicing near my old office. It is now over twenty years since I started handing out those cards. We stepped into the exam room he uses for consultations. This physician nodded with his head toward a wall cabinet next to where he always sits. He didn't say anything. As I stepped closer in that direction I saw taped on the side of the cabinet one of my old business cards. It was there as instruction for all his patients.

When I gave one of those business cards to patients, often after they had been operated upon, it was the usual like, here's my number so you can call me. In so doing I waited a moment then asked them to turn the card over to see what was on the back. Almost in direct proportion to how serious their illness had been, or continued to be, a patient would spend a certain amount of time reading this list of suggestions. Some looked at the card they held for a very long time. This was not conventional nor expected. This is not what doctors do...such people were evaluating everything in a new light, based upon what was happening to them now. They were thinking.

If I were still in the "business" of surgery, I still would be handing out those cards. The only one on the list to modify is the third. Now I would say, ACCEPT YOUR SELF, emphasizing three separate words and leading up to the fourth recommendation. This is an esoteric point. You may see it only as a play on words, but as I continue to learn I say, differentiate "your self" from the yourself that is in most people's usage. Throughout this book, when I have felt a reminder of this is in order, I have tried to use the two words, not the one. Your Self turns attention inward to the essence of who you are, where it needs to be.

This idea explains the perennial popularity of the movie "The Wizard of Oz," though the movie is almost 70 years old. The characters accompanying Dorothy all want something: a heart, a brain, some courage, and are following her, going somewhere, to get fixed. The wizard, charlatan that he is, shows enough resourcefulness to tell them what they seek already has become manifest in their actions. They already have it! He gives each of them a symbol of achievement. The same is true for Dorothy. She just wants to go home and that is within her power as well.

What we are talking about is not the outer being everyone sees. It is not what is around you and everyone calls reality. What you have within you may be, at this moment, the only thing over which you can feel you have any control. So start there. Be conscious of defining who "your self" is. And certainly, for all the things that you may be feeling remorse about right now, you need to forgive and accept who your self is first of all.

So this brings us up to the time Renewal got started. I hope this chapter has explained more clearly why this came about. I also hope I have given you more understanding of things that made a young surgeon develop the way he did. The events in this chapter, and others like them, were the things that bent the branch that grew to be my life. This has been some of what I see as bending me in a different direction. It moved me into something more meaningful in my personal and professional life. I have come in an unanticipated direction. When the idea to start Renewal for education and more in-depth conversation with patients came about, I felt ready.

In the next chapter we will look at some of the people who were attracted to similar work. They have helped immeasurably in making Renewal successful. Then in Chapter 8 we introduce you to other physicians who have thought about concepts, and done things, you need to be acquainted with. Some have written books that are listed in the back as part of Renewal's recommended reading. This is the journey of understanding the dimensions of your personal opportunity for renewal. It is the way toward healing that presents itself with every cancer.

A few more things before the next chapter: I want to emphasize that a personal odyssey once begun need not end. After I started Renewal and saw it come to fruition, I kept learning. You will too. In the 1990s I started having headaches and bouts of dizziness. I remember the headaches, almost always originating deep in my right ear, felt like someone driving a railroad spike into the side of my head. The dizziness was episodic but sudden in onset. It could cause me to stagger and grab something to avoid falling down. I thought this was due to overwork and not getting enough sleep. I didn't know what to do about it. Self-diagnosis is always a mistake but it took a long time for me to overcome my obstinacy and get medical advice. It turned out I had an inner ear problem and fluid buildup in a tiny confined space that was causing both the pressure pain and dizziness.

My symptoms did not respond to medication or months of inactivity and rest. When I finally came to realize the potential danger to patients of my operating and being subject to these spells, I decided to retire.

This problem with vertigo or dizziness has caused physical helplessness at times. For a time I was depressed by a sense of loss over my surgical career. Still, in retirement I have achieved a new balance point. Life still allows me to do many things. I continue with Renewal as it has evolved. Along with my bout of hepatitis twenty years earlier, this new illness increased my empathy and helped me identify more closely with the issues at Renewal. New doors opened and I continue to learn from these illnesses, just as you, the reader, can learn from yours.

If you have felt terrible, felt weak and helpless, have worried about losing your job and if you are going to die, I feel I understand. This is the common experience, not the exception. You can help your self and you can seek out others to learn the value of mutual support.

Another event I want to mention as part of my post-graduate education did not occur until 2004. In October of that year my wife Maureen had an abnormal mammogram followed by surgery for breast cancer. I have seen thousands of women for breast problems and performed surgery on many of them. This time, in the most important relationship in my life, I was relegated to the sidelines. I had to watch as someone else took care of the surgical part. Maureen had been a visitor and helper at Renewal for years; now she became a full-fledged member.

In the postoperative period Maureen chose to undergo a course of radiation. I volunteered to accompany her to the radiation center each day for her treatment. After the scariness of the first one or two sessions, she said she was fine, there was no need for me to keep coming along. I was trying to call on all my past experiences and be the best support I could. "I want to come," I told her, "I'm not doing this just for you—I'm doing it for me!" And it is true I wanted to feel as involved as I could be. I think the reality of her breast cancer brought us even closer. And, at that moment, I knew I finally would be writing this book about Renewal.

In early 1981, after concluding a three-year stint first as Chief of Surgery, then Chief of the Medical Staff at my hospital, I planned a six month adventure traveling around the country. We just took off in a motor home—my whole family. Each morning we sang along with a Willie Nelson tape about being "On the Road Again." That could be another long story, but for brevity I'll just say that my practice partners were dissatisfied with the arrangement. They prevailed upon me to come back after four months and get to work. There seemed to be a worry that I wasn't ever coming back. I remember thinking that was odd; I loved my surgical practice and was approaching the top of my game. I often made a habit of telling people I planned to practice surgery as long as I was able.

The reason I mention this is that one of my friends, an older primary care physician in the community, was very insistent upon my return that he and I go to lunch. So as soon as practical, I went to his office and we did go out to eat. I was uncomfortably aware my friend had been keeping his eyes on me since our first sighting that day. This scrutiny continued all the while I was relating the travels I had made with my family, most of it in that motor home. Finally I became self-conscious enough to ask, "Why are you looking at me that way?"

Without moving his gaze he said something about how I looked good. He could see that I still had all my hair. By then I know I looked puzzled, so he explained, "Well, the word got around the hospital that you had cancer. While you were gone everyone said you went someplace for special treatment."

So, be aware personal growth is not a spectator sport. When you start to change you are likely to be misunderstood. Someone once said if you want to be loved you should talk more about your faults than your successes. I am trying to do that here. This business with cancer is new and different. You still can be open and honest, but only you can judge how much to share.

Another thing I want to add about continued learning is what is shown on the following pages. It is a reproduction of an actual drawing I made on April 17, 1985. The date is obscure but is in the upper right-hand side. It was part of the idea of creativity in self-analysis I was following for Renewal at the time. This methodology of diagramming did not originate with me, but I like using it. The idea is to take some problem, something of importance you need to understand the ramifications of, like cancer, and let your mind free-associate with that idea. It is one of the devices you can

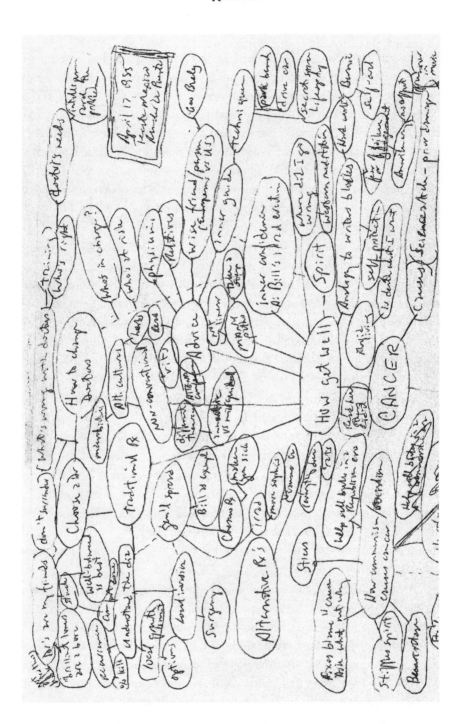

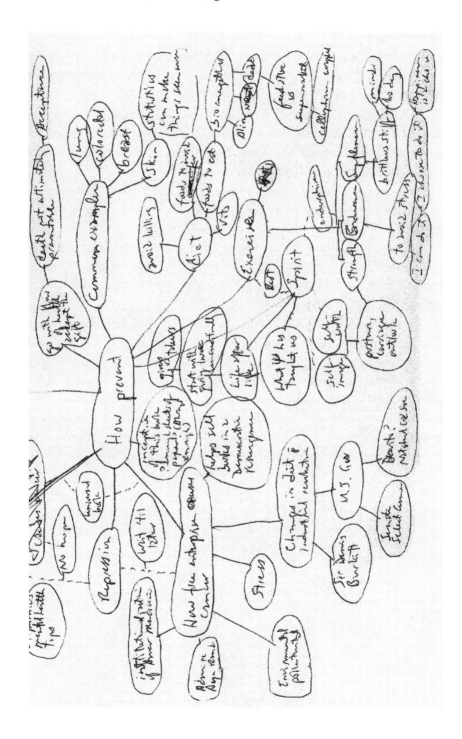

use to pry the lid off your subconscious. Using my exercise as a template may help reveal the blocks and conflicts that disturb you. It may help make connections you have not considered yet. It also can reveal solutions your deeper self is processing and wants to offer up.

So what I did, in this context of Renewal, was start with one central idea, cancer. Well, as the thinking started to move along, what is important to me about that? I put a few items down. Each addition led to another level of association, and that new level to another.

Take a look then try it from your own viewpoint. Your ideas about cancer may be very different from mine. Where this exercise takes you is the important part. At some point be sure to start naming names. Draw real people into your concept and see where they have relevance. Like a similar exercise of tabulating positive elements in your life in contradistinction to negative ones, see which people and activities you associate with certain ideas.

Remember where this is coming from. This is not a cosmic message from outer space beamed to you through the fillings in your teeth. This is coming from inside you. The inner you is trying to break to the surface and may be carrying an important message. Spend time analyzing, trying to understand clearly what you are saying to your self with an exercise like this. Thomas Carlyle (1795-1881) once wrote, "Our main business is not to see what lies dimly at a distance, but to do what lies clearly at hand." All that is required is being honest and persistent. Try it.

CHAPTER 7

PEOPLE WHO GAVE US THEIR GIFT ────────

> *"If you want others to be happy, practice compassion.*
> *If you want to be happy, practice compassion."*
> — *Dalai Lama*

Renewal was primarily a success story reflecting the lives of its members. Around the members was another group of individuals, the ones who came to share their unique blend of knowledge and experience. Over a span of years this became a large and diverse collection of people. Some of them were physicians, some nurses or psychotherapists, others dieticians, social workers, or physical therapists. All of them had developed beyond the conventional boundaries associated with their professions. Others, like yoga and Tai chi instructors, music and dream therapists, ministers, Native American medicine men, healers of other sorts, volunteered their time to come and meet with Renewal. Some had health issues of their own to temper their outlook, some did not. Many who came as speakers identified with us and considered thereafter that they too were Renewal members. Overall their thinking and resource diversity had profound effects. Our book is not a survey of all such diversity, but this chapter will give you a sampling.

As he explains below, Dr. Staples came to our community to serve in a dual role as hospice medical director and as a specialist practicing medical oncology. He met with Renewal many times and was always a favorite because of his kind and empathetic manner.

— Russell Staples, MD —

When I came to Evergreen Hospital in 1991, I was aware that Dr.

Claude DeShazo had a group for cancer patients called Renewal. I assumed it was similar to a variety of cancer support groups that I had been loosely involved with for years. I was a medical oncologist/hematologist and had been in this specialty for about 10 years. In addition I had been hired as the Medical Director of Evergreen Hospice at that time. I knew Renewal was one of the meetings that took place at the Hospice Center, so in that sense, I felt a responsibility to facilitate a number of meetings with this group. But I did not really understand what it meant to facilitate a group. When I was there I would lead the group, talking about some subject or another. From the viewpoint of my expertise in medical oncology I provided information about some new treatment, the failure of some old treatment, a description of a particularly vexing problem around cancer care, or something about terminal care that I found interesting.

When I was first introduced to the group, Claude did it, and I was in the position of listening. I saw myself responding with sophisticated comments anytime a group member asked a question. I was fascinated to see Claude had a great comfort with silence. He would come, welcome people to the group, and then we would have a time of checking with folks. Everyone reported on their progress along the road to wherever they were going. Claude did not seem concerned with having control over the subject matter. The next thing I learned about the group was it wasn't about the techniques of cancer care. It was about members' feelings, questions about physicians and nurses, comments about how irritating individual physicians could be. I learned a lot. This began a change in me that was much needed. I was starting to listen.

I also learned about more holistic ways of treating cancers, things other than the standard ways of cutting them out, radiating them to the point of non-viability, or treating with chemotherapy (which was a way of poisoning them). I heard first hand about what people had to tolerate with all the side effects to the bowel, the bone marrow, the sense of well-being. Some of this was unproven methods, but I was beginning to appreciate the value of story. With my training I had accepted the randomized, double-blinded clinical trial as the gold standard by which all treatments were compared. I still think they are helpful. But I no longer discount any of the other ways of treating cancer patients that are helpful. I know that treatment in the medical sense is only one part of how lives of folks with cancer are impacted.

I have come to see that observing the whole picture, treating not just the physical aspects of the disease, but also the spiritual and emotional aspects is important. I became a better listener. I began to hear from patients the many issues in their care we left unaddressed. I listened to the many ways an individual could be helped, and they were all different. For one person it had to do with the physical aspects of the disease. For many people the spirit or emotional things eclipsed the physical. This was another of those instances where I had the opportunity to listen and learn. I still felt an urge to teach something, but I was becoming more of a presence. Instead of teaching something, I could just be. Instead of sharing something of importance that I just had learned, I was discovering the ability to listen, really listen to others. I saw this was a lesson Claude had learned some time ago. That leads me to the next leg on my journey.

In 1995 I suffered a stroke. This was a dissection of the left middle cerebral artery. It carried a very ominous prognosis, about 50% mortality in the first 48 hours. It was a Thursday morning. I was dressing for work when I suddenly collapsed and fell to the ground. I did not realize what was happening to me. I had lost the strength on my right side. I did not have any control over that side of my body either; I could not speak. The very thing I had always been so facile and confident with, my speech, was suddenly gone. My son found me on the floor. He called my wife; she called the neighbor, and also my best friend, then finally 911.

I remember two things about the experience that day. I remember being in the emergency room. The director of nursing came into the most emergent of areas in the emergency room to find me. She started talking to me and I was thinking, "I don't want her to have this conversation with me!" I knew at that point I could not speak. I wanted her to get out of there, but did not have the ability to tell her that.

I also recall waking up in the middle of an angiogram. I looked up at the monitor and thought, "I could make my own diagnosis—that's a blocked left middle cerebral artery!" I felt a certain peacefulness about my stroke. I wasn't worried. I knew I would survive but I had no idea of the kind of survival it would be. There would be time enough for me to deal with all the grief.

I experienced an act of kindness that first night following the stroke. One of my friends, the director of hospice, came into my room about 10 p.m. She asked if she could sit with me. She would hold my hand and remain quiet. She stayed all night until early the next morning. I slept fitfully but I was aware of her presence. I understand why I felt uneasy about the ICU and CCU in general. They were horrific places where there was no room for any privacy. After six days in that horrendous environment I was overjoyed to be moved to a private room. I had made substantial improvements in both my speech and strength by that time. While I was getting my first real shower I began to weep uncontrollably. Some of that was because of the hyper-emotionality caused by strokes. Part of it was the beginning of my deep depression.

Days later I was just beginning my first rehabilitation session in the hospital when a physician colleague popped his head into my room. He asked in a cheerful voice if I minded having a group of four medical students come in and examine me. I did not know what to say. I was confused about how to say anything so nodded my consent. The experience was utterly humiliating. I needed to learn how to say 'Hell, no!' That would have been so much healthier for me.

I had one other instance when I wept. It was a Saturday morning. The nurses were upset about short staffing for that shift, and the energy everywhere was tense. I had a visit from a woman elder from my church. I burst into tears. I do not remember anything of what she said to me. The fact she let me cry was better than all the platitudes she shared. I look back remembering the value of simple presence. It was of greater value than any words that might have been said.

The stroke began a journey through a time of depression for me. It lasted a couple of years. I am thankful (I think) that I did not have pills offered to modify the nature of what I went through. My wife Janet said that while on vacation six months after the stroke I was so withdrawn she could not imagine how we stayed married. Miraculously, my wife and children always treated me with love and respect. I do not know why. I always had the sense that they cared deeply about me.

Professionally I went through a hard time. I had to adjust to the fact that I would never be the same. I held out the fantasy that I would be different, but still adequate, and still functional. I had the sense that I knew all the facts that I had learned in medicine, I just did not have the ability to express them. I saw only loss. I saw change as a series of deficits. I did not have any context to see the blessings of those losses. I do now. I could see my thinking alter as I went through the months of rehabilitation. Time marched on: four, five, six months. I wanted others to see that I was making improvements and progressing. Instead my physician colleagues and hospital administration lost patience immediately. I came to the conclusion that I would have to close the practice portion of my career. The administration of the hospital became very cold to me. Even my colleagues in oncology section made changes in our interactions that were very hurtful. One woman administrator even changed her mode of speaking. When she approached me to speak she shouted. Did she think I had sustained a hearing loss? She was only too glad when I agreed I needed to leave my position as Hospice Medical Director and close my oncology practice.

The odd thing about the transition was that I was also part of the interview process. I had to interview every candidate to be my replacement. Claude treated me with respect and thoughtfulness. But, for others it was different. One of my physician colleagues, who was a friend from a previous position, said she could not imagine the sort of changes I would have to make professionally to prove that I was insurable. It finally sunk in. I needed to leave the whole thing professionally and start fresh.

I left Evergreen Hospital. I did not do anything for three months. I kept my license, barely. Then one day I got a call from Rodney Smith, a person who I had interviewed once for another position. He now was the director of Hospice of Seattle. He wanted me to interview for a job in downtown Seattle, as co-Medical Director of his hospice. I explained I did not have a practice and was not expecting one. He said that John Herseman an oncologist from another hospital was functioning in half of the position. He thought I would be a good candidate for the other half. I interviewed for the position and got the job. That was the beginning of a seven-year relationship that was very productive and nurturing. I also did a quarter of continuing pastoral education. I started a path toward a masters in transforming spirituality at Seattle University.

I am now a chaplain at a different hospital from Evergreen. I do a small spiritual direction practice two days a week.

What have I learned from this journey? First, change is inevitable but it does not have to be the enemy. Change does lead invariably to a liminal space. Liminal refers to a kind of space that is unknown and uncertain. It is not a comfortable place. That is possibly the most creative place for a person to be.

Second, and very personally, I believe that nothing happens by accident. The deficits I experienced with the stroke were the very ones I needed to learn lessons from. I lost 15% of my spontaneous speech, but I learned the art of listening. I lost some of the strength in my right hand. I learned to write slower, but much neater. I would never say that I love my stroke. I loved my life as a medical oncologist and Hospice Medical Director. Those interactions with patients as a doctor were holy and precious.

Third, it takes time. Thirteen years have passed since my stroke. I started to get over the depression in years two and three. This second lesson, the one about listening, came to me at year five. It has grown and is still growing. New lessons keep coming and teaching me new things every day.

LISTENING
— Gerri Haynes —

This is one of the wisest women I know. She met with Renewal many times and guided the conversations. She was fully capable of serving as facilitator and in exploring sensitive issues with empathy and understanding. She had one life as a critical care nurse specialist, followed her heart into hospice work and served for a time as Clinical Director of our local facility. She went on to work with a local children's hospice and with mothers who have lost children. She has been President of Physicians for Social Responsibility and has traveled the world providing for people in need. In addition to being wife, mother, and grandmother, she has had her own experience with cancer. All these careers (and more) blend into an extraordinary experience. I asked Gerri to comment on some of what she has learned.

Listening carefully to one another was the norm in Renewal. Compassionate listening is a hospice class I have taught for many years. Listening is one of the greatest gifts human beings have to offer. An English hospice director, Dr. Peter Kaye, wrote, "Listening is more than waiting to speak." These words form the basis for guidelines that help a listener open his or her heart and hear more clearly. Too seldom do we listen without waiting to speak. Too often we are distracted by the formulation of what is to be our response. We are seldom aware of the mirror of self we present to speakers addressing us in our conversations. It is essential that we do understand our role. Listening is communication at the most loving level. Imagine the stories that follow if listening hadn't been happening:

"This woman is driving the nurses to distraction – she's on her call-bell every 30 minutes wanting pain medicine. They're giving her as much as they safely can, but she's not getting relief. I think it's something besides physical pain. I'm her surgeon, not her psychiatrist. Will you come to visit her?"

That's a call I took one day in my work. No psychiatrist either, I hung up the phone and called the ICU nursing station. Was this a convenient time for me to visit? Permission being granted, I first closed my eyes and spent a moment preparing to listen. Then I walked over to the ICU. I knocked on this woman's hospital room door, asking permission to enter. I walked to the patient's bedside. I introduced myself quietly and simply, "Your doctor has asked that I come to visit with you and see how this hospitalization is going. Is that OK?"

"Sure", the woman responded without looking my way.

"I could be here for as long as 45 minutes. Is that OK with you?"

"Sure", the woman replied, again without looking.

"May I sit near you?"

"Of course." This time she glanced at me.

I pulled a chair close to the bedside. I leaned close, placing my heart below the level of her heart, ready to listen and receive anything that flowed out. I began with, "Would you tell me how you are doing?"

A window began to open between us. For a moment there was just silence, then the woman looked down at me. She shifted in her bed, turning to better see me, "I've been in this hospital for two weeks. I don't seem to be getting better."

I remained silent for a moment then asked, "Have you ever been here before?"

"Yes"

I didn't say anything and after a moment the woman continued, "Last year, about this time. I was here with my husband. He had a terrible disease. Our three children and I sat in that waiting room down there for hours and hours. The doctors couldn't seem to stop the bleeding my husband was having from his intestine. He got whiter and whiter and weaker and weaker."

I could see from the woman's face that talking about this was getting harder.

"My children—they're all adults—were impatient with me." she continued, "'Can't you do something?' they kept asking me. I didn't know what to do. We prayed. Our minister prayed with us. The doctor was trying. Finally, he came into the waiting room and said, 'Your husband is still bleeding. We think it might be slowing, but it hasn't stopped. His blood levels are very low. We need to give him some blood, or I'm afraid he won't pull through this.' My children shrank back from this doctor guy..."

The woman paused for a moment, then went on, wanting me to understand, "We're Jehovah's Witness – we don't take blood – it's against our faith. So I walked this doctor out into the hall and asked him, how much time do you think he has?"

"'If we don't give him blood today, I think he won't live through tomorrow.' That's what he told me. I paced the hall by myself. What could I do? He was dying. I prayed for an answer. We'd been married 40 years. He was my life. About half an hour later, I phoned the doctor back at his office: If you give him blood, do you think he might live?"

"Well, there's no guarantee, but for certain, if we don't give him blood, he will die very soon."

"I'd already made up my mind, Give him the blood, I told him."

This was increasingly difficult, but she went on, "That night, I barely slept. My children wouldn't speak to me. They thought I had condemned their father to hell. He got the blood. Then, the next day, he died. My children haven't spoken to me since."

She wanted me to understand her life as it was now. "I wander around the house, wondering what else I could have done. I've talked with the doctor; he tells me he'd have made the same decision. But he's not a Witness. He's not one of us."

I was silent again for a long minute, then I leaned even closer, "How long have you been ill?"

"This started about six months ago," was her reply. "First I missed a few days of work, and then I missed another week. Finally I went to my doctor. He told me I needed this operation. Away we go, I thought. And so I'm here," she concluded with resignation. "But I'm not getting better. And now I'm alone."

Her conversation continued, talking about her own life, her husband again, her family when the children were young. She wept some of the time. She switched to talking about the things that still give her strength: friends, her faith, getting exercise. We had been together for about 45 minutes. Finally she had said everything and was quiet.

I thanked her for talking with me. I didn't offer any commentary. I did ask if I might visit again the following day. "Oh, yes, please," the woman sounded relieved. As I rose to leave she reached up and pulled me to her in a hug. She held up her right hand, asking that I wait a moment. With her left hand she began probing her abdomen as if checking something. Surprise wrinkled her face. "You know," she said, "when you came in, I was about to call the nurse. Right then I had more pain than I could tolerate. But...now..." her voice expressing surprise, "My pain is gone!"

Listening is more than waiting to speak, just as Dr. Kaye said. Our listening helps give the speaker access to his or her inner counselor. It is their chance to process before the mirror we give them. It provides a way to approach the questions and the answers that are being held within.

Woody Allen said, "Eighty percent of success is just showing up." When we show up for each other and listen, our presence can be a powerful gift.

"Please come to visit the woman at the end of the hall." began another phone call. "She's dying, barely able to talk. Her husband is afraid she doesn't know what is happening."

I went to the ward and toward the room. As I spoke to the nurse caring for this young, terminally ill woman, her husband came out the door.

I took another step forward to get closer to him, explaining that if he was willing, I would accompany him back into the room. I would help determine what his wife knew about her illness.

Even though the husband was with me I knocked on the door and waited a moment before going in. The wife lay quietly in the bed. She did not acknowledge our presence. I approached her bed, introduced myself, and followed saying I would like to speak with her for a few minutes. The young woman opened her eyes for the first time and silently nodded yes with her head. "I'd like to sit in this chair next to your bed," I continued, as I came closer to the bed, "May I hold your hand?" I got another silent nod. Her husband crossed to the other side of the bed and picked up his wife's left hand.

"Can you tell me what is happening with your disease?" I inquired.

Nothing happened at first. Then the patient replied, speaking very slowly, "I feel like it's raining down...raining down all over and I can't wipe it away." She paused then said again, "Raining down."

I asked her, "What does this mean to you?"

She absorbed this for another long moment then said, "I guess it means that I can't get well." That was her understanding. "I'm not going to get well. I'm going to die."

I noticed that the husband was squeezing her hand tightly. His tears began falling onto the sheets. Again, quietly, I probed some more, "Are there some things you need to do before you die? "

"Oh, Yes!", she suddenly was emphatic.

I responded with, "This might be a time to tell about them."

Very slowly, she itemized several things that were worrying her. She turned to her husband looking for his response. He bent closer, "You and I can talk about those things. We can take care of them."

I excused myself, feeling I was no longer needed.

Listening, waiting, trying not to anticipate any answer, these are the things I use. Listening, one person to another. As humans, this is our gift to someone else and to ourselves.

After these examples here are some suggestions or guidelines for you to consider:

1. Make an appointment before meeting.
2. Set aside your other concerns and any concept of how the interview will go.
3. Respect privacy. Knock before entering the room of the person to whom you will listen – even if you can only knock on a separation curtain!

4. Identify yourself, even if the person knows you. People in pain often have lapses in remembering names.

5. Say why you are there. Ask if this is still a convenient time (something may have happened since the meeting was arranged, making this time now inconvenient).

6. Suggest a time period you will stay. This gives framework to either a short or longer conversation and confirms the allotted time will work for both of you.

7. Ask if you may sit nearby. It confirms that you have committed to having a dialogue.

8. A heart-to-heart conversation means you make sure your heart is not higher than the heart of the person to be heard (lower is better for receiving).

9. A simple question like, "How are you doing?" may be the only question necessary.

10. Listen without interruption and allow long silences to develop. This can help the speaker clarify for him/herself what they want to communicate.

11. Avoid asking clarifying questions to draw out someone's feelings as we normally do. It is more respectful of the speaker if you don't inject yourself into the conversation.

12. Interruptions require the speaker to evaluate your words. If you are silent you allow the speaker to prepare for going deeper.

13. Avoid telling of your own experience. Not now. This is the speaker's time.

14. Thank the speaker (physical touch may be helpful) to complete the time together.

15. Avoid over-evaluating the conversation as you leave or even later. The speaker will be doing this and may tell you at another time about the effects of the conversation.

It is possible to listen compassionately on the telephone. To do this, set aside any distractions and really listen. If you don't interrupt the speaker he or she may stop to ask whether you, the listener, are still present. But by not interrupting you are allowing the speaker an uncommon opportunity to sort through questions and problems. Doodling, playing computer games and the like are distractions even if you aren't being seen. Give the gift of your full presence.

Listening is also possible with people who are in coma. All of the guidelines above still apply. In addition, when you come near a comatose patient, still ask permission to touch a hand/elbow/shoulder. Then, pause before doing so. Following the patient's breath with your own breath or commenting upon any facial/hand/leg/foot movements you see may increase communication. In their deeply helpful books on coma, Arnold and Amy Mindell teach us our presence with a person in coma can help that person complete their work — to process the final tasks of their life and have a peaceful death.

Marie's family had grown tired maintaining a vigil by her bedside. They had moved to the far corner of the room and sat visiting with each other. The nurse, Vicky, told the family, "I think Marie is not in pain. More medicine doesn't seem to be needed. She's been in this coma for nearly 10 days. Would you mind if I tried to reach her by breathing with her?" The family readily agreed. They all moved closer to the bed to see what would happen.

"Marie, it's me, Vicky, your nurse. You've been here in the hospice for nearly two weeks. I'm thinking that pain medicine may not be what you need just now. I'd like to breathe with you – to come as close to you as I can." The nurse paused to let this be absorbed. Then she began the process of "breathing with." Each time the patient breathed, the nurse accompanied with synchronous, audible breaths.

Within five minutes there was a change in the room. Marie appeared to relax and even looked more aware despite her coma. Her eyes were still closed, but she seemed to be less "deep." Vicky, sitting near the bed, said quietly – in timing with the breaths, "Marie, it seems that you will not live many more days. Do you know this?"

In a distant yet distinct voice Marie responded, "Yes." The family moved even to the bedside, variously touching her hands and legs.

Vicky: "Do you know that your family [and gave their names] is here with you?"

Marie, Very slowly: "Yes."

Vicky: "Is there anything you need to say to them?"

Marie, again, very slowly: "Yes"

Vicky: "This might be a good time."

Marie, with painstaking clarity: "I....love...you."

The family stayed close to Marie's bedside for the next eight hours. Marie remained peaceful. She did not speak again and gradually stopped breathing.

Listening offers us incredible gifts. Waiting to speak brings us the love and wisdom of our shared humanity. The members of Renewal were great listeners.

DECISION MAKING
— Gerri Haynes —

Gerri Haynes has another bit of wisdom to share. This is a decision-making process she has adapted and refined for years in her own work. As you will see, this had some unanticipated value in Gerri's own life.

When we listen to each other we can assess what decision making is possible within a person's value and belief systems. If we do that medical choices become more clear and peaceful. The choices made also become more authentic. Members of Renewal discussed communication challenges frequently. Some of these challenges were with family members and some with physicians. The work of Jonsen, Siegler and Winslade presents a model of ethical decision making. Their work is a pathway to creating a common language in a new conversation. What they did creates a communication pattern capable of removing barriers. This model has assisted thousands of patients and their family members in making difficult choices.

Renewal members recognized that communication between professional caregivers, patients, and families can be complicated. Many things get in the way: lack of speaking candidly to each other in the past, the shadow of new fears, and cultural or spiritual differences. For the medical professionals there can be a reticence to communicate information when its meaning or outcome is uncertain. As information is passed among patient, family and professional caregiver, the intent of the original speaker can be lost. Cultural language, that language within a family's culture on one side and the arcane language of medicine on the other, can present challenges in understanding. While listening to information presented by the medical professional, a patient's anxiety and fear in the moment may block understanding of what choices are available. The professional caregiver may feel time constraints or lack comprehension of the patient's history or ability to understand. All this may diminish meaningful dialogue. At the same time lack of listening may cause the professional to misunderstand their patient's needs or goals.

With the use of an organized, replicable pattern for decision making, understanding between patients, families and professional caregivers can significantly increase. When we comprehend correctly and communicate honestly, all parties in the conversation are assisted. We reach decisions that lessen the pain of an illness. When we communicate well, it is a joy.

In their textbook on clinical ethics, Jonsen, Siegler and Winslade present a framework for discussion of ethical problems. Often called "The Four Box Method", this has been expanded to form a model both for clinical discussion and medical treatment planning. The original four boxes are: Medical Indications, Patient Preferences, Quality of Life and Contextual Issues. These are enhanced by clinical history, documentation of discussion and a plan of care. Their model provides a pathway for understanding. It helps patients, families, and professional caregivers to better understand each other and formulate a plan of care that fits the patient. Here is an explanation of how this works:

In the model, identified problems or symptoms are listed, along with options, potential risks, and benefits for treatment. These are the Medical Indications. For each option, the patient expresses preferences such as: Do I want that treatment? Are the potential risks to me worth the possible benefits? Are there things going on in my life that make greater risk more reasonable or less reasonable? Are there other people I want involved in my decision making? Do I have an over-riding preference such as, Do Not Attempt to Resuscitate! Or, Try any treatment available! Or, is what I want something in between? These are the Patient Preferences.

Under Quality of Life, the patient lists what he or she loves in life. What gives him or her pleasure? What does he or she like to do? What gives value and meaning to the patient's life? In the fourth box, the Contextual Issues, all the mitigating circumstances of the patient's life are noted: family members, where does the patient live, does the living place offer impediments to care, are there spiritual or cultural beliefs that will affect care, is care coverage by the patient's health plan a concern?

When patients and families and medical professionals take the time to discuss these areas, a plan of care gradually emerges. Having a facilitator present can help. The facilitator is someone to organize and document the discussion. In this way current issues receive priority. Such a methodical approach helps when attention shifts to long-term decisions and consequences. They appear less ominous.

People with long-term and progressive conditions find this Four Box process particularly helpful. Its structure provides a method for recognizing and detailing incremental changes in their condition. Parents of children with progressive illness use this model to track subtle differences that affect care decisions. Some patients, having used this process for their medical decisions, go on to use the model for other major life decisions. These include career decisions, purchase options. One young mother said, "I use the model for everything, even buying my groceries!"

As a nurse consultant, I have used this model hundreds of times. I use it with patients and with my friends. Then, I finally had the opportunity to use the process for myself.

One Friday night, while getting ready to go to sleep, I discovered a small lump in my right breast. My husband is a physician. He is always calm and unflappable, but in this instance he was disturbed. He saw this lump as an urgent problem—getting the lump removed needed to be done! For me, a quiet and peaceful series of events unfolded.

I was 58 at the time and a diagnosis of breast cancer was not shocking. My mother died at age 48 after the cancer in her right breast had metastasized to her liver. Early death for women in my family was almost an expectation. Fifty-eight was already old for me, I thought. During multiple visits to bombed areas in Iraq, I had spent time in some of the most polluted air on the planet. I lived and still live in the Seattle area—known to be the highest breast cancer region in the U.S. Breast cancer is an epidemic and having lived "so long," I did not feel alarmed or frightened by the diagnosis. There were treatment choices to be made, though, and I wanted to find the treatment that would best fit my beliefs and needs.

At that time, I worked as a consultant at Children's Hospital in Seattle, managing a Robert Wood Johnson Foundation Palliative Care Grant. In this grant, we utilized the decision-making model explained above. I had adapted it to plan and coordinate patient care. The model is simple but can be time-consuming to complete. Somehow knowing that seemed to honor the solemnity of the decisions to be made.

My breast biopsy and lymph node dissection was completed by a general surgeon who is a good friend. I remember he treated me with great kindness. With all the test results in hand, I met with a breast cancer specialist and a radiation oncologist. I also talked with other oncologists I knew and with family members to discuss my thinking about the choices available. Then I filled out the Four Box model and reviewed it with those who had helped me. For me the results looked like this:

History of Present Illness

Generally healthy, active 58-year-old. Discovered lump in upper R breast 4/21/00. Last mammogram 18 years prior. Mammogram and ultrasound (4/24/00) suggestive of R breast malignancy. Surgical biopsy of mass (4/24) revealed high nuclear grade/high mitotic rate infiltrating ductal carcinoma (1.5 cm mass with infiltration to surgical margins.) Consultation with radiation oncologist 4/27 re radiation therapy options. Excision of breast tissue surrounding biopsy site and full excision of R axillary nodes 4/28. All surgical margins and nine of nine nodes demonstrated no evidence of carcinoma/neoplasm/malignancy. Consultation with UW breast cancer specialist 5/2/00. Review of pathology and treatment options. Further pathology examination of full tissue mass from breast revealed no evidence of ductal carcinoma in situ and no evidence of infiltrating neoplasm. On 5/6, stumbled and caught self from fall by extending R arm. Tearing sensation followed over next six hours by formation of hematoma filling R axilla and extending to R chest. Rx with needle aspiration (partial), pressure and oral antibiotics. Fluid again collected in this space over the next twenty four hours, leaking through puncture wounds, but repeat attempt at needle aspiration was not successful.

Medical Indications

Surgical excision: Complete

Follow-up therapy. Assuming complete removal of the presenting cancer, there is a 25 – 40% risk of recurrence at the site and 10-12% risk of cancers in other sites of the body.

I. Mammogram in three weeks to confirm surgical removal of branching calcification seen on 4/21 mammogram.

II. Radiation: 28 treatments over 5 ½ weeks, beginning 3 – 4 weeks following surgery, with a 5-treatment boost to the site.

A. Benefits: Reduction in the 25-40% risk of recurrence at the site to 2 – 7%. (60 – 75% of women who receive radiation therapy do not benefit from this treatment.)

B. Risks: Arm swelling (?%), radiation pneumonitis (0.2% - although Dr. Einck at UW states he has never seen this without chemotherapy), fatigue, damage to chest wall muscle, sarcoma (0.05%).

III. Tamoxiphen: Five years oral

A. Benefits: 40% reduction in the 10-12% risk of cancer at other site – making the risk of other site cancer 6-8%

Patient Preferences

Avoid further medical treatment if at all possible.

I tolerate medicine poorly and have a relatively high tolerance for physical discomfort.

I prefer not to take medicines into my body – the idea of radiation is alarming to me, as is the possibility of five years of daily pills.

I want to make a responsible decision about further treatment and hope to learn all I can about risk/benefit ratios for available treatments.

Medical Indications	Patient Preferences
B. Risks: Headaches, hot flashes, depression, thrombophlebitis IV.Chemotherapy: A. Benefits: 30% reduction in the 12% risk of cancer at other site or 9%. When using Tamoxiphen therapy, adds another 5% benefit to the potential benefit of Tamoxiphen (45% of 12% = 5.5%)). B. Risks: Many – most known to me V. Close follow-up with mammograms of R breast q3months for first year, q 6 months for five years and yearly after that. VI.Hematoma: observation and evaluation	

Quality of Life	Contextual Issues
I love my life I love • working and playing with my husband, children and grandchildren; • being with friends, • working on the stuff of my conscience – serving in places I love, • digging in the dirt, • walking on the beach, • exercising, • hiking in the mountains. • reading, • laughing. Except for the commute, there is little about my life I would change. I am blessed.	Live happily with my husband, Bob, and our dog, Ignatius. Often, others stay temporarily in our home. We have six children, four children-in-law, six+ grandchildren and several informally adopted children. All of these people are remarkably healthy. We are active. Spirit is important to us although we go infrequently to an organized church. We endeavor to live what we believe. Bob is a physician and has assisted in obtaining medical care quickly for me – as have the physicians with whom I work. Bob and I love spending time with our family and have formal and informal ways to bring us together regularly. My only living extended family: a brother in Portland, two half-sisters and one stepbrother. They are well. My mother died of breast cancer more than 50 years ago. My father died following a heart attack more than forty years ago. No other family members have had cancer. I work three days/week through a State contract and a Robert Wood Johnson Foundation grant as a pediatric palliative care consultant at Children's Hospital. Much of

Quality of Life	Contextual Issues
	my time is spent as a volunteer as a lecturer, grief counselor, and as the vice-president of Washington Physicians for Social Responsibility. I have traveled to Iraq three times in the last two years – a toxic environment. In the past five years, I have occasionally (rarely) seen an acupuncturist and a massage therapist for treatment of back pain. I do not regularly seek medical care.

Discussion

In reviewing this rapid process, I am aware that I am on a steep learning curve re breast cancer. It seems to me that I am dealing with relatively small percentages in this decision-making. The 100% chance that I will have to spend hours of my life in relationships I do not want doing things I find unnecessary (horrifying but not frightening) tends to lead me away from any further treatment for the cancer that has been removed. I hope to live long enough to see all of my children enjoying their children. I do not want this time injured by medical care that may not be essential.

Plan

Action	By what date
Continue reading and evaluating treatment options	Ongoing
Repeat Mammogram	May 24, 2000
Follow-up visit with oncologist	TBS (after 5/24)
Follow-up visit with radiation oncologist	TBS during May

Based on the JSW Clinical Ethics Model

Completing this simple outline helped me to articulate my primary goals. Surgery had removed the cancer – I had protective treatments to choose. This form was sent to the oncologist who had recommended treatment. Although I did not hear from her and did not see her again, it helped me make decisions that were in concert with my goals. I completed my medical care with a course of radiation and am well.

In the intervening years, I have continued to use this decision-making method in many settings. In our culture (Western US) reflective decision making seems not to be a focus of education. With the use of this model, a pattern of organization for making decisions that can be transferred to reflections on other decisions is a welcome benefit.

In my story, at the completion of treatment, a local feature writer told the story of my treatment for breast cancer – the story appeared in the Seattle Post Intelligencer. The medical professionals I had visited were understanding of my choices to varying degrees. Some understood I wanted to protect myself from just going with the numbers, basing my care only on statistics. Some were more thoughtful about seeing the higher percentages of cure as positive and supported my choice to not accept chemotherapy. Following the publication of the newspaper article I received calls and notes from hundreds of women who either were related to someone who had breast cancer or had cancer themselves. All wanted to talk about treatment decisions and coming to a choice that was a fit for them. This structured process outlined above helps in sorting through choices. It has helped many women reach decisions regarding their own care.

Some of the times I met with the Renewal group we studied this method. Similar to my day job, pediatric palliative care programs across the United States have also used it. The original method, the Jonsen, Siegler, and Winslade ethical decision-making four boxes, continues to be in use. Medicine owes its originators gratitude for creating this framework for assisting clinical decision making.

— Sally and Michael —

Somewhere, I don't remember the source, I read a version of this story from the Far East:

The Lord said to Moses, "Why did you not come and see me when I was sick?"

Moses replied, "I didn't know you were sick. And besides, you're God; you don't get sick."

Then The Lord said to Moses, "One of my dearest devotees, someone you know, has been ill. If you had gone to see him, you would have seen me."

What follows is a personal account told to me by a woman friend who for many years was a gynecologic nurse practitioner. She had a very busy and successful practice. She was not directly associated with Renewal so this story is one of the rare exceptions in this book. On the other hand what she related was very helpful to my understanding. I think you will learn from it too. It is a first-hand experience of one person helping another and what can happen when that change begins to take place. This is Sally's story.

The day I met Michael he was so cute and easy to talk to, and I was very nervous. He was the husband of a partner of mine at work. She worked in our medical clinic and he was a 49-year-old geriatric physician. I knew that much about him from her, but he and I had never actually met. Michael had developed a degenerative, fatal illness of his own and was now housebound. What he had carried a nasty name: Multiple Systems Atrophy. I never heard of it. It is rare, a debilitating brain atrophy that is uniformly fatal. As the brain shrinks, all the body functions weaken. Michael was housebound in bed or a chair with very limited mobility for the last two years of his life.

I am an Advanced Registered Nurse Practitioner. I have been practicing since 1973. My two sons are grown. I had traveled some, but in addition I was looking for some community service work to do. Nothing really got my attention until my nurse friend at work told me that her husband was ill and unable to work any longer. I think the subject came up because that was the weekend she had to go and move his things out of his office. The things that cause Michael to be housebound were vertigo and weakness. He was unable to read due to the vertigo. He was too dizzy to take wheelchair rides outside, or even leave the house. He watched very little television. Michael and his wife had no children so when she went to work he was alone. She put in three full days a week at our OB/Gyn office. She told me that Michael had a cell phone and a life alert call button around his neck. He could transfer from a chair to a scooter if necessary and was able to talk and think clearly.

After hearing this story a number of times I asked my friend if Michael could use some company. She said she would ask him. Michael said yes, even though he and I had not met. His wife and I had alternating schedules, so my plan was to go visit Michael on one of my days off when he would be alone.

The wife and I met for lunch one day and set up a date that I would start my visits. We were just going to see how it went. Neither of us had a plan for the future or had any idea how it was going to work out. My intention was just to help out a little if I could. That was the humble and simple beginning of one of my greatest personal journeys.

As the first day for a proposed visit approached, I started to get nervous. What were we going to do? I hadn't thought about that. I asked my friend and we decided I could start with reading Michael medical journals. He couldn't read due to his vertigo but wanted to keep his medical skills up to date and his brain active. As I progressed through that work week I had some challenging clinical cases come up. I didn't fully understand what was wrong with several of these patients. So I decided I would get second opinions from Michael while I had this internal medicine physician as a captive audience.

Just prior to arriving I called Michael on my cell phone to be sure it was still a good day for me to visit. I drove on to the house and let myself in with the key the wife had given me. As I opened the door I called out, "It's Sally."

I found Michael sitting in a lounge chair, waiting in silence for me to arrive. It was a little scary for us both that first visit. Neither of us knew what to expect. I came in with my thermos mug of tea and feeling apprehensive. There I was, armed with a few medical journals and some questions that I had about those patients of my own. We said, "Hello, how are you?" to each other. He thanked me for coming and added, "Nice to see you. Now what?"

Luckily, I have the gift of gab. I think I just started in with, "Well, I guess I can pick your brain with some medical questions that have been coming up for me." I remember those first 4 or 5 visits were under the pretense of my picking his brain of medical knowledge and my reading medical journals to him.

We quickly became closer friends. My intended 1-2 hour visits turned into 4-6 hours visits. It never crossed my mind that I probably exhausted him. We both seemed to pass away the time, just talking. Each week we became closer. Our conversations turned into intimate exchanges, with me talking about my children and my problems, my future trips, him always asking me questions about me, work, the kids. A plumbing accident caused my house to flood; we talked about that. From time to time he'd tell me about the effects of his illness and his worsening condition. At first we ate lunch together but soon after I started coming he declined to eat with me. He said he wanted to lose some weight. He was getting weaker and it was getting more difficult to transfer himself from chair to scooter to bed. I wanted to take him for wheelchair rides, car rides, whatever I could think of to distract him. He declined saying that all of those things made him more dizzy. There was practically nothing medically I could do for him.

What I gained from this relationship is nothing I anticipated. Originally, it never even crossed my mind that I would benefit; I was just trying to be of some help. Over time I realized Michael was steadfast in his example to me. He showed me how to accept things that are not fair, accept things that cannot be changed, and how to maintain dignity in a situation that was mostly hopeless. He was gracious to me as a guest in his home. He was always in the moment. I have never before or since met anyone like that. He was so accepting. Such acceptance was, and still is, a new concept for me. Being a mother, and a nurse, and a child of an alcoholic, I had spent my entire life trying to "fix" everything.

For me, up until recently, I led my life anticipating the future. That gave me a sense, but a false one, of order and predictability. I was the type of person who lived by the clock, made my lunch the night before, made dinners for the rest of the week on my day off, and had a calendar of upcoming events that always was crammed full. Yes, I had a good time, but I was living in the future. Michael had no future. Yet he seemed at such peace for that entire year I knew him. I still don't understand how this wonderful man arrived at this place of acceptance. His wife told me he was like that when she met him, some 20 years earlier. She told me he first caught her eye when she went into a dying man's room to be with him. Michael was sitting there when she went in. That's when the two of them met. She was the nurse and Michael was the geriatric physician. They separately had concluded that no one should die alone, and this man was alone. Each of them had been sitting with him off and on when they had a few moments but had never met. That was the beginning of their relationship.

A few times Michael and I got on the subject of his funeral services. I will never forget his attitude. He said, "I won't be there." So he wanted it to be entirely left up to his wife. He felt she was the only one who would know what she wanted when the time came. He trusted her to do what she thought best. Michael said he had no needs regarding service or memorials. When the time did come, she had a small home service.

One day when I was showing him pictures of a hike I took up Cathedral Rock in Sedona, Arizona, I told him, "It was my body and my eyes up there, Michael, but I tried to exchange energy with you. I visualized that your eyes were in my head and that your eyes were seeing this stuff in the pictures."

It was as simple as that when I took my trips. I took pictures with him in mind and when I returned from Sedona again, or from South America, Michael and I would go over the pictures. We'd discuss the sounds and the energy that surrounded the two dimensional photographs. He seemed to really enjoy the stories. His only regret, he told me once, was that, "I wished we'd traveled more. But now that I am so ill, it isn't possible."

Our last visit was Christmas of 2006. I was home for Christmas for a visit in the middle of a 4 month sabbatical to South America. We spent several days together, Michael and I. He was always encouraging me about my travels. He laughed at my stories and enjoyed the travel e-mails I sent from different places. Two months later I was in Pucon, Argentina, one of the most beautiful places on earth. While there I received an e-mail at an internet café. Michael had died, his wife by his side. She wrote me that he had just slumped over and died. She also wrote that even though she knew this was coming, now that he was gone, there was a lot of grief to handle. Michael died one month before his 51st birthday. I thought of that and flashed back to his 50th birthday when I had been included in the small family party 11 months before. I had given him some videos, mostly comedies. Michael said he enjoyed listening to them even when it bothered him to watch the screen.

The wife's message was a hard one for me to receive. I remember I stumbled back to my little room at the boarding house where I was staying in Argentina. I was a long way from home but that day I began a new phase in my relationship with Michael.

Originally, I was drawn to Michael because I thought he might be lonely. I thought I could be helpful. I went to distract him from his physical decline, to cheer him up, help pass the time. My visits did keep him occupied, we even laughed some. My thinking was, to fill in, and keep him from loneliness. But Michael never once mentioned he was lonely. He was not angry, he was not wishful. He was thankful. When I recall all this now, I think I was lucky enough to have been in the presence of someone that enlightened.

The night Michael died I had my first long heart to heart talk with the moon. The next day I took a very long, very high hike into the mountains. I was alone but I felt Michael's presence. He was very calm there with me, too. Sometimes I visited beautiful old cemeteries asking for wisdom from the dead. That trip to South America I sat on exposed roots of an 800-year-old tree. I asked for energy and felt I received it. I moved around to lots of places finding in nature I discovered the most peace. At a lake, on a ledge in the mountains, deep in the forests, at the cemeteries, watching the butterflies, swatting at flies, listening to the birds, things seemed to be in order. The more simple the questions I asked, the easier the answers came.

Soon after this experience Sally retired from clinical practice. She increased the amount of time spent in new traveling adventures to full time. As this is written she is currently on her second extended trip to India, studying and traveling alone.

— Jonathan Collin, MD —

Dr. Collin practices and maintains two local clinics. He is one of the resources in our community that donated his time to come and meet with Renewal. He gave updates to the members on developments in his area of expertise, complementary medicine. Maybe we don't have to clarify this, but Renewal members constantly were searching for practical, concrete information. Though it may seem otherwise to you after reading earlier chapters about the benefits of our close association and bonding, members wanted to learn things they could take home and use.

Dr. Collin always got the Renewal group excited because he shared information about alternative medicine. This was information most members couldn't get anywhere else. This field is currently called Integrative or Complementary and Alternative Medicine, or CAM, but the label isn't very important. Like his visits with our group, what follows is a chance to give you the sum of one practitioner's experience over thirty years. It includes Dr. Collin's suggestions of how a cancer patient should view themselves. It is how to proceed if a person wishes to explore alternatives to the conventional treatment course they are contemplating or have already tried.

This report is based upon interviews I did with Dr. Collin over a period of several years. Jonathan started out sharing with me how he got started. He was going down a path of conventional internal medicine residency when he wandered into a conference on orthomolecular and integrative medicine. He recalls the episode as almost an accident. That one experience changed the thinking of this physician-in-training and served to redirect his subsequent career path.

The story of what's new in complementary medicine will change from year to year. Such information can become outdated and so is not what I want to present here. This, rather, is about an approach. Dr. Collin is qualified as few others to provide this information. For 25 years he has been Publisher and Editor-in-Chief of a periodical he founded called *The Townsend Letter for Doctors*, now titled *Townsend Letter* (for more information, go to www.townsendletter.com). One of the monthly issues each year is devoted to reviewing alternative therapies for cancer and makes for highly informative reading. Dr. Collin defines his area of practical experience this way: "I practice quite differently from the present-day Cancer Centers. People who see me have either been treated conventionally already and want to know what else is out there, or, they have already made a decision to take their diagnosis outside the conventional system (surgery, radiation, and chemotherapy). They usually have a diagnosis and a protocol given to them elsewhere (staging procedure, treatment)." Here is a concise summary of Dr. Collin's observations about cancer patients based upon his practice, followed by some advice:

- People want to find a mechanism, or reason, or something in their environment or experience that will explain their disease process. Supporting them in this search, or notion, is important because doing so in and of itself tends to help them get better.
- Some people are not interested in conventional approaches and want another approach.
- With cancer the patient and I need to embark on a course of exploration about the options.

- For the person wanting to explore alternatives, go to someone with experience in the alternative field. Do not try to change the thinking of the doctor you have now.
- For starters, you need to find out the true prognosis of conventional therapy. Being told that chemotherapy is "standard" for this or that diagnosis is not enough. If the answer you receive is that conventional therapy has less than a 50% success rate, in my opinion, that alone is sufficient reason to immediately open yourself to alternative medicine.
- Try some mind/behavior process even if it is only group counseling. (Getting people to do this is a bigger barrier than you might think.)
- Get involved in some educational process. The problem here is, at the beginning, being overwhelmed with books, videos, etc. The information available about alternative medicine has increased by at least ten fold. It's easy to be shot-gunned by so much material. There may be 10,000 books and articles available now. So, either be guided by a practitioner or do a very focused search engine query.
- Better to see someone locally than take off to some exotic clinic for treatment. Even when staffed with good, experienced people, clinics abroad tend to gravitate to two or three philosophies about therapy. They tend to crowd every patient into one of those few chosen regimens. Start with some basic things like vitamin C, other vitamins and minerals. B-12 is a particularly important component of healing. Other things he recommends are fatty acid supplements, specific immune support and dietary measures [here it is very difficult not to lapse into making specific recommendations].
- Similarly, there is a transition in conventional care going on right now that is hard to evaluate. Not necessarily bad, just hard to evaluate. Cancer care is now a big business in this country. A large amount of money is flowing into it. Compared with even five years ago, mainline institutions, big hospitals and clinics, are adopting integrative approaches to improve their marketability. At least six naturopathic schools in the U.S. and Canada are training physicians dedicated to CAM cancer practices. Specialty training in naturopathic medicine includes a discipline of naturopathic oncology. This is greatly different from the allopathic medical oncology specialty with which most people are familiar. The number of practitioners in this field still is small, but there are adjustments being made in how cancer treatment is planned and executed. Hospitals allowing alternative therapy to come into the fold after such a long period of resisting it are an interesting phenomenon.
- Deciding to go with alternative therapy is a major decision. Dr. Collin

estimates only 20% of those with cancer consider it. Of these, maybe a fifth will elect one of these proprietary therapies [i.e., one of the specialty cancer hospitals or clinics, here or abroad]. These institutions are very expensive in the treatment they give, not the least of it being the travel involved and the likelihood that insurance will not pay for it.

- There are many other approaches advocated originally by some individual who may no longer be in practice. Their treatment concept only survives in some publication or isolated clinic. A journalist named Patrick McGrady (now deceased) for several years provided an analysis of a person's pathology report and test data. For a fee, he then made a recommendation about a practitioner specializing in that particular disease process. He did this on the theory that people were best served by seeing a special, extraordinary doctor for most types of cancer. There are a few others who provide this type of clearing house service. Ralph Moss has written several books and has a directory on alternative cancer therapy. On a more general level the basic healing process was covered by Norman Cousins in his book, *Anatomy of an Illness*. Drs. Alan Gaby and Jonathan Wright are also experienced individuals that Dr. Collin knows personally.

- Then, at some point, the patient and the practitioner need to agree to make a decision.

- Dr. Collin says he is aware that alternative cancer therapies pose great uncertainties. This is especially true at the moment when the patient asks, "And what do you think the outcome will be?" If a patient completes chemotherapy and radiation and does poorly, someone may say the practitioner was responsible. Or, at least the doctor feels some sense of failure. With alternative medicine the practitioner worries that a poor outcome will be blamed on the administered alternative treatment and failure to complete conventional therapy.

- At least it is easier to gather information. Just out is *Cancer Recovery Guide: 15 Alternative and Complementary Strategies for Restoring Health* by Jonathan Chamberlain. Also look for *Alternative Medicine Magazine's Definitive Guide to Cancer*, 2nd Edition, by Lise Alschuler, ND, and Karolyn A. Gazella. Both books describe an integrative approach to treat cancer.

— Kimberly Mathai, MS, RD —

In an earlier chapter Virginia Brown was mentioned. She was the person who met with Renewal repeatedly in our early years to discuss nutrition. From time to time other nu-

tritionists including dieticians working with cancer patients as a specialty met with the group and shared their approach. This field has become much more scientifically based in recent years. Kimberly Mathai is another person we were fortunate to attract as a speaker. She has her own nutrition consulting business in Seattle, Nutrition by Design. She speaks on this subject frequently and has written The Cancer Lifeline Cookbook (Sasquatch Books, 2004). She can be reached at kjmathai@nutritiondesign.com.

What follows below are some of Ms. Mathai's observations and general recommendations to us. She accepts that most people undergo conventional treatment, so she approaches the subject in terms of what additional things a person can do. There is additional material in the final chapter and Appendix on diet at the end of the book. Fortunately for everyone, The American Institute for Cancer Research, with funding from World Cancer Research Fund International, presented and published its findings after a five-year review of scientific findings (November, 2007, Washington D.C.). The conference title was "Food, Nutrition, Physical Activity, and the Prevention of Cancer: a Global Perspective." The title is a mouthful and the published report heavy reading. But for anyone interested in fact-based information, that report can be very helpful. For now at least, that report provides the most comprehensive evidence-based judgments and recommendations. Here, as if she were presenting to Renewal, is a summary from Kimberly Mathai.

- The question is, what can nutrition do? This is not exclusively about prevention; it includes cutting down on recurrence among survivors.
- What is mostly animal, slightly vegetable, and the same over and over again? The answer: the American diet.
- The most important thing is to get to a plant-based diet. Fill at least half your plate of food with color *(What Color is Your Diet?* by David Heber is a good resource). By this I mean specific colors, like blueberries. Purple color vegetables and fruits contain cancer-protective compounds called anthocyanins. Orange for carotene is another example. Ideally your plate is two-thirds vegetables, fruits, grains, and beans with only one-third animal protein.
- What is a whole food? Answer: something you can grow. Also, is it organically grown? What has been done with it since harvest? How many ingredients does it have?
- Plant-based foods have antioxidants and phytochemicals. Most cancer-causing chemicals enter the body as procarcinogens. Cytochrome P-450 is a family of enzymes produced in the liver that make these DNA-damaging substances water soluble so they can be excreted in the bile or urine. This is phase I of a two-phase process. In phase II other enzymes break down compounds that are not completely detoxified in the initial process. All of these enzymes, especially in Phase II, can be augmented by dietary components that aid in destroying

cancer-causing substances. So, eating the proper foods can both help protect and repair our systems.

- Where do we get antioxidants? From the plant-based foods with bright colors mentioned above. Others come from foods with strong flavors and pungent odors such as onions, garlic, herbs and spices. Vitamin E is important in this regard and can be obtained from nuts and whole grains.
- Plant-based foods contain thousands of phytochemicals. Some of these serve as antioxidants to protect cells from damage. Others, like selenium, act to prevent cancer. All this can be viewed from either the phytochemical side or the cell process side. Knowing the chemistry is not so important; it's the cell processes that are important.
- Get 30-40 grams of fiber each day. Only 10% of the U.S. population does this. This translates into eating six to eight servings of vegetables and fruit each day. A serving is defined as half a cup or about a handful, so that really isn't such a large amount. Beans (legumes) also are an excellent source of fiber.
- People already know they should have fruit and vegetables; most just don't know how to do it. So the question is, how do I get the proper food in my diet?
- Dietary change does not have to take a lot of time. The food industry is helping us here. We can get the basic things in pre-packaged food like frozen vegetables or a bag of baby carrots, for example. If necessary, create options like a food delivery system instead of going for crummy take-out fast food.
- How do you manage food in your life? Well, if you've learned to be successful otherwise in life, you know you need to set goals, like having a meal plan.
- Shop locally like a farmer's market and eat local foods. We need to develop a relationship with food. Other cultures have a different relationship with food: elsewhere people shop every day for fresh ingredients. They take what they purchase home and make their food. After eating a meal they take a walk.
- Nourish your immune system: fiber supports 60% of the immune system. Fiber absorbs noxious materials in our GI tract. It also propels waste products and toxins through the gut at a faster rate so we can eliminate them from our system more quickly. We have an entire gut-assisted lymphoid system. The liver both manufactures essential nutrients from what we eat and detoxifies procarcinogens we ingest.
- Vitamin D is a very important nutrient. It is hard to get from foods and

if we don't get enough sunlight, we can become deficient, especially in cold or cloudy climates like the Pacific Northwest. People with a normal level of vitamin D are 60% less likely to get a number of common cancers. This is something that can be checked with a blood test by your doctor.

- Eat "good" fats. There are three types of dietary fat. Most saturated fats are solid at room temperature and come from animal sources. Hydrogenated oils are artificial fats used to extend the shelf life of manufactured foods. This is the trans- fats you hear being condemned. Trans- fats promote heart disease. Avoid them. Unsaturated and monosaturated fats like avocado, canola, and especially olive oil are the "healthy" fats. Essential fatty acids are important to the diet. They can be obtained from plant sources such as flaxseed, pumpkin, soybeans, and walnuts. Good animal sources are fatty fish like salmon, sardines, and mackerel. Omega-3 fats act as anti-inflamatories and may help prevent a number of chronic diseases like arthritis.

— Maria McKinney, D.M.A. —

Beethoven supposedly said he left his music to heal the world. There is much practical interest now in how music can be used to lessen acute pain. Dr. Maria McKinney has made a lifetime study of the therapeutic value of music. She came to Renewal to help our members gain some appreciation of its uses. In her talks she emphasized the need for attunement to specific needs. She shared information from her Casa Maria Research Center (which has since closed), and from her book on the subject, The Healing Tones of Music. *Some of the material below is excerpted from that work, but Maria also recently summarized her work for inclusion in this book. She currently can be contacted at maria@music-massage.com.*

In recent years there has been an increasing interest in the mind-body connection. Scientists have discovered that negative attitudes (criticism, resentment, anger, timidness) affect certain cells and organs of the body which then manifest disharmony and dis-ease in the physical body; whereas positive attitudes (love, forgiveness, peace, faith, patience) promote healing in the body. As one listens to music of the Great Masters, negative attitudes can be transformed into positive attitudes...particularly when the music is heart-felt. My interest in researching Classical music (see *Healing Tones of Music*) was to discover ways to promote positive attitudes for healing purposes. For example, selections of music composed by Wagner – with its long melodies – can lessen fear and bring stability. The music composed by Beethoven can transform a lack of faith into more joy. Forgiveness, gratitude and hopefulness are powerful tools for healing.

My interest in healing also turned to a recording *(Musical Massage Sound Therapy)* of two ancient Gregorian chant scales. These scales are constructed in such a manner that the vibrations from the long tones bring harmony and balance to the energy centers and unite the higher self (eternal self) with the physical. The intent of this recording is to help hospice patients make their transition in a peaceful manner. For example, my sister, caught up in grief after being deeply hurt by her husband, manifested colon cancer – which was diagnosed too late for medical treatment. How to help her? She began having much pain, so she listened to her choice of choral music and *Musical Massage Sound Therapy.* Her family was amazed that she miraculously was spared all pain after that and made a peaceful transition.

—m—

Maria also mentioned in her book the fact that our bodies react to sound and musical vibrations just as they do to other stimuli. Music can raise or lower the heart rate, raise or lower body temperature, alter breathing patterns, and affect the autonomic nervous system. Psychologically music can be used to help in the creative process. It can strengthen the immune system, stabilize moods, and bring hope and peace. It can bridge the finite across to the infinite. Her book contains a chart of most of the best known composers categorizing their work as affecting either the physical, mental, or spiritual being. She also has a section characterizing therapeutic effects of various instruments including the harp, violin, and flute.

As mentioned above, Wagner exhibited fear while Beethoven had a deep sadness and aloneness. Wagner's music was therapeutic for his own ailment and for those with paranoia and fear. Beethoven's music is helpful for those with a poor image of themselves.

Maria explains that each of us, and each cell within our bodies, vibrates in harmony with certain sounds and certain colors and lights. A person wishing to take advantage of such a discipline needs to maintain a positive attitude and develop healthy habits such as are outlined elsewhere in this book. A person can benefit from seeking out someone with experience in this field. Fortunately degrees in music therapy are becoming more common at colleges and universities. A therapist needs to be both intuitive and sensitive to the needs of a potential client.

In addition to Gregorian chant, one of the earliest music forms, Maria points out more recent ages of music. In the 16th century, part of the renaissance, much liturgical music was written. The influence of the Church was strong and included guidelines dictated by the Council of Trent. It was a time of well-known sculptors, painters, and craftsmen and known as the Spiritual Age of music. Music from that time strengthens and allows creative energies to flow freely.

The baroque music of the 17th century is referred to as the Aristocratic Age. It was more instrumental than in the Renaissance time. Composers were hired by the nobility or the church. There was an extreme contrast between the wealthy and the poor. Baroque music is soothing, balances the body and mind, and is uplifting to the soul. The most therapeutic music from this period was written by Bach, Handel, and Vivaldi.

In the classic and romantic periods of the late 18th and 19th centuries composers became independent and were no longer hired by the nobility as before. Many were idolized as performers, not just composers. This was a time of growth for the middle class and is referred to as the Heroic Age of music. Its theme is largely flowing, colorful melodies. Musical instruments and voices were used with great imagination. The music of this period was either dramatic, meditative, descriptive, and/or emotional. It helped people identify more with self, group, or nation, or with nature and creativity. The great masters of the period had high spiritual awareness, sensitivity, and intuitiveness. This is the time period most often selected in music therapy work.

In the 20th century music had great diversity and is referred to as the Chaotic Age. Therapeutic music uses Gershwin, the musicals by Rodgers and Hammerstein and others, and early jazz. Some of the music of this century was decidedly un-therapeutic with dissonance that causes stress and unmelodic music that gives no direction. Maria feels some harmonies bring fear and weaken us with harsh electronic sounds, loudness, and addictiveness. She feels the composers reflect the consciousness of the people! At its best the New-Age music of the 1980s reflected a more peaceful time and put the whole being together. This is music for those who need to expand, to go beyond the limitations of the present experience, and at the same time receive a grounding or sense of being centered.

— Robin Maynard-Dobbs —

Robin is one of the people who educated Renewal in using other expressive arts in healing. Others talked about disciplines such as dance and physical movement which are not being covered here. Robin's background was in painting. When we updated our connection recently she told me, "Once a person makes a drawing, it is very powerful if they can look at it and say, 'I am what I have just drawn.' It lets that person (or client) see outside what's going on inside. It is self-actualizing.

"This is not learning how to draw," she continued. "It's how to make the connection." Like some others interviewed for this book, Robin has changed her emphasis as the years passed. She now spends more of her time with women and their weight issues rather than cancer and similar illnesses. She can be reached through her website. Here is more of what Robin related to me about her earlier work and its value.

Robin's mother was an artist. She encouraged Robin to take a sketch book with her everywhere she went. Robin remembers she never got bored making sketches as she grew up. In college she was an art major and got involved in batik and making all sorts of banners. She became interested in both texture and color and this led her to spend a year and a half in Paris. While there she learned a new technique of painting on silk. She especially remembers viewing "The Hand of God" at the Auguste Rodin museum while in Paris. She was so moved she wept.

She began producing for arts and crafts shows and launched her business in 1984. She found it difficult to support herself with painting and later switched to working with clay. She liked the fact she could begin a work without knowing what form would emerge from the clay. She found this to be very visceral; memories of the past often surfaced. She began to depict what those memories were in clay and connect to them. To her it was almost like becoming a child again. She also kept drawing (pastels were her favorite medium) and started taking out her contact lenses when she drew. "I'm so blind I could barely see what I was doing without the contacts," she explained about removing her visual aids. "That way the art took over and moved me." Only after the initial sketching was over did she put her contacts back in and finish the work: "It was only then I saw what I had done."

Around 1991 Robin became interested in art therapy. She took course work and later worked as a mental health therapist and counselor. It was during this time Robin met with Renewal. She explained her work and the principles advocated by authors in a number of books. She gave us a reference list of a dozen books including Betty Edwards' *Drawing on the Right Side of the Brain* (1989). In our present conversation Robin updated her recommendations with three additional books for any reader. For an introduction to the subject she likes: *Painting from the Source* by Avida Gold, Harper Perennial (1988); *Art and Healing* by Barbara Ganim, Three River Trust/Random House (1999); and *The Creative Journal* by Lucia Capacchione, Swallow Press/Ohio University Press (1979).

Robin feels a person with cancer approaching this field for help needs to realize books she recommends are not about learning how to draw or paint. "You can get that elsewhere," she says. What she teaches is a skill to interpret the outside world we live in by taking an interest in a person's inner world. Look at anger: what color and shape might anger have for you? How big do you see it? Can you use pastels to depict that? A variation is to ask if you can visualize an emotion you have as an animal. If you can, what animal is it? Can you put that on paper? Robin says if a person is intimidated by trying to draw, she tells them to scribble. "Scribbling seems to be less intimidating."

Robin goes on to say, "Show me what your energy is like. Ask yourself, 'Where am I right now?'" Then, "Draw what it would look like if you were whole." Where would you begin? Robin added, "I often give a client a very small piece of paper. It's easier if they don't think they have to fill in a lot of space. Often the client will have their own image of themselves. I say to them, what does that look like?" So, small paper, pastels (because of their vividness and texture) and, scribble!

Since the time with Renewal, Robin has moved on because of an interest to work with women. She came to appreciate the pervasiveness of eating disorders and wanted to do something to help. She is now an eating awareness facilitator. "A lot of women are not connected with their emotions," Robin told me. "Drawing can let women like that [and anyone else] discover a deep connection to the miracles within." When she meets with groups Robin shows them her own work [some of which is on her website]. She has women in these groups start by drawing hunger. She has them do a dialogue with their stomachs. It helps them access their feelings about food. "If they say they can't draw, I tell them just to put color on the paper...let the energy express itself. This can tap into amorphous feelings and help them become more clear by seeing what they have put on paper. It lets a person do something that is immediate and then, for them, it becomes alive." Robin can be contacted at robin@awareeating.com.

— Christy and The Pacific Institute —

This final section in Chapter 7 requires three separate introductions. It also brings forward the opportunity for the reader to pursue more specialized knowledge by familiarizing yourself with educational opportunities at The Pacific Institute. Their website (www.thepacificinstitute.com) states in one place the organization "...teaches people how to manage change, set and achieve goals, lead more effectively, and think in ways that create success." It has many avenues for exploration.

The Pacific Institute was founded in Seattle in 1971 by Lou and Diane Tice and they still lead the organization. Lou's work began as an outgrowth of motivating students when he was a high school coach. Diane has been his partner in developing what has become a sophisticated and world-wide educational institution. About 22 years ago she developed a serious form of cancer. This illness provided an opportunity for her personally to test their beliefs. Her story is available on the website and provides a number of her insights.

I met Christy through a surgical patient of mine. One afternoon she was visiting in the hospital while I was making rounds. What makes her memorable is the personal story she related to me late that afternoon, standing out in the hospital corridor. At that moment Christy was a thirty-something widow with two young sons. The boys were just reaching school age as I recall. Christy was strikingly attractive and gave the impression of being sweet and soft-spoken. She told me her husband had been an airline pilot. Their prospects as a couple with their sons were good and they were very happy. Then the husband developed a leukemia-type cancer.

"He didn't try," Christy said in recalling his unwillingness to fight the disease, "he just quit!" Her husband lived only a matter of months after diagnosis and had been dead for about a year at the time we spoke. The emotion spilling out with her words caught me by surprise. I still can see her fingers curling into fists and hear the anger causing her voice to crack, "He just laid down and died without a fight. He left me with these two boys to raise all alone!"

When I learned Christy had been through The Pacific Institute's program and was a volunteer speaker for their alumni group, I asked her to come to Renewal. Her presentation was a combination of videos featuring Lou Tice and her commentary, plus a bit about her personal encounter with cancer. Diane Tice has been good enough to review what I have written and update material with the Institute's current thinking and approach.

Several years later Christy met someone and remarried. She moved and I lost track of her, but this is the introduction she gave Renewal to The Pacific Institute philosophy.

The Pacific Institute teaches the concepts of self-image psychology. There is no limit to what can be accomplished in all areas of our lives. One place to start is with "Possibility Thinking" about the imaginary limits we set for ourselves or others set for us. What can we change? What are we locking on to in our thinking and what might we be locking out? If we can just change the way we think we can change the way we act!

How do we think? The mind has three parts: Our conscious mind perceives, evaluates, makes associations, and decides. Our subconscious mind is a data bank that handles automatic functions. The third part, our creative subconscious, maintains our individual sense of reality by making us act like the person we see ourselves as. We say things like, "I'm terrible at remembering names" or, "I'm good at math."

Our self image is the sum of all the attitudes and opinions we have stored in our subconscious. It is built from our own self talk and the 50,000 times a day each of us engages in the thoughts we have about ourselves.

The subconscious does not judge what is real versus what we imagine. It just stores everything. The only way to overcome a negative image is to block it out with a self-imposed positive thought. Words really do have power over how we act!

The subconscious acts like what used to be called a servo-mechanism. When I use clear pictures with emotion it is the same as creating, or re-creating an event. Once you create a belief about yourself, you will act like the person you believe yourself to be. We have to eliminate belittling thoughts and sarcasm; such things demean what we want to be.

We want to be happy and have a successful, useful life. We move toward what we think about, so focus on what you want, not on what you don't want. The essence of this is controlling our self talk. We need to make our self talk intentional. Use of words like, should, could, would, can generate guilt. Avoid using them. When you mess something up, say to yourself, "That's not like me…" And correct the mistake with, "The next time…"

We humans think in pictures. The subconscious has images and feelings, but has trouble getting a picture of a "don't" or a "can't". Our subconscious carries out what it is programmed to do, dropping the "don't" in messages we give ourselves an imprinting of the remainder. If we keep going over negative things, reliving them, they eventually make us sick. Once a speaker at Renewal told of a woman friend with no obvious infirmity being confined to a wheelchair for years. According to that speaker, this friend had a habit of beginning every opinion she expressed from her confinement with, "*I can't stand…*" How many times have you heard someone say, "I'm sick and tired of this!"?

We have to create the picture of what we want just like a sculptor chipping away on a block of marble already sees the image of what will emerge. If you see someone perform an objectionable act, skip berating them for what has happened with a "don't". It's better to counsel them with, "I will not tolerate your behavior; I see you as…" and inject a positive image. Remember to <u>intend</u> to be loving in what you say.

We behave according to the "truth" as we see it. We strive to stay in a comfort zone we create. When we get outside that comfort zone, move above or below that self image our subconscious pictures us as, we create a negative physiological reaction: palms sweat, our voice cracks, pulse races, etc. If we are content and comfortable, we won't be motivated to change and to grow. We won't use our potentials. It benefits us to broaden our comfort zones.

My subconscious doesn't care about my potential; it is trying to fulfill my internal picture. Disorder is upsetting, but when we put everything in order, creativity is shut off. To reach our potential we must leave this sense of order behind. Create constructive imagery, not constrictive imagery.

We are usually told to do something not for the good, but to avoid the bad. This is coercive motivation and always has an "or else" attached to it. When I feel I have to, my subconscious resists the coercion. When I'm pushed, I push back. The subconscious protects me from coercion either from outside or from within. When do I say, "I have to?" What I see as "have to" is external, an outside force trying to control my life. And when I say, "I have to" it gives permission to say, "It's not my fault!" to whatever happens.

High achievers don't push themselves with "have to." They wait until they want to do something, then they act.

Figure out what you want to be. Stop using circumstances, family, and finances as an excuse. The motivation has to come from within me. It needs to become "I cause..." what I want to happen.

Visualization is the tool for improvement; combine visualization with affirmations. First visualize a goal. Make it as vivid and detailed as possible. Think, how would I feel if I were to reach the goal right now? Think future tense as if it has already happened.

Then create the affirmation. To be effective, an affirmation must be written out, must be personal, must be stated in a positive way, and it must be in the present tense. Write it as though the goal is already a fact: "I feel healthy, happy, and full of energy." Or how about this one: "I am my own expert, and I am not affected by the negative attitudes and opinions of others." An affirmation must be written as an achievement with no comparisons. Use action words, exciting words. Use accuracy and balance. Temper your statement by being realistic.

This kind of affirmation needs to be read, visualized, and felt with your eyes closed for 15 minutes twice a day. Do this upon awakening and upon going to bed. Some people write affirmations on Post-its and stick them on the bathroom mirror. What you write needs to have intent and spirit behind it, something important to your well-being. It generally takes one to three weeks for this process to take effect.

This section may sound like a concept you have heard in some other situation or it may be entirely new to you. Even with the caution above about being realistic, such bold assertions may seem beyond you, especially if you are contending with cancer or just feeling miserable. If so, take another look at Nancy K.'s story in Chapter 2. See how she made use of similar ideas. And again, take time to explore The Pacific Institute's website. With further study some information there may appeal to you.

Renewal

CHAPTER 8

HEALTH PROFESSIONALS IN THIS WORK ————

This chapter introduces you to a number of physicians who have done important work in explaining the principles of self-healing to the public. They have either done research or explained scientific findings in ways the average reader can understand and use. I came to know most of these men as a part of my search for the best information for Renewal. I talked to them while in the process of writing this book. Several of them became involved with Renewal over the years. They interacted with the group or came to town to participate in events sponsored by our group.

Several others, like Dr. Jonathan Collin, Dr. Staples, and the psychologist Dr. Luke, were geographically close to Renewal. For that reason their contributions were placed in earlier chapters. At the end of this chapter are two additional physicians I know only through their work. The exposure to all these pioneers is brief, but it will serve to round out your experience in reading this book. When you see something applicable to you, read more from that person's books or go to their website.

I will briefly put this in context. Collectively much of the work in this chapter has been done outside the mainstream of American medicine. For too long patients could not get much useful information from physicians on how to involve themselves and further their own interests. Things are better now but I cannot say too strongly that without the work of the men in this chapter, and others like them, Renewal would not have been the vibrant collection of people it is.

Information hard to obtain is one thing. Lack of effective communication between physicians and patients is another. Over the years we heard hundreds of anecdotes in the Renewal meetings about the encounters group members had with their physicians. These often were emotionally charged, high-stakes interactions. The majority of stories were about unsatisfactory experiences. That is a fact, but not our central message.

Understanding was missing. Both the lay person and the medical professional failed to comprehend what the other was trying to say. It takes two for a dialogue. What did each have to contribute? The medical practitioner is a fount of knowledge. In the case of some subspecialists what issues forth may be limited in scope, but it's there and available. A recent survey of patients with serious illness revealed between half and two-thirds said their physicians never had a candid discussion with them about issues. Some patients may have gathered a considerable amount of information from the internet, reading, and family history, but what is the best way to use it? The question for the patient should be, "How do I maximize this moment?" The physician needs to challenge his or her self constantly about how to be more effective in presenting advice.

Part of the problem is the seriousness of the conversation. When people are anxious, just like when they are mad, they don't listen well. Renewal members usually had longstanding relationships with a primary care physician. This was someone they knew and trusted before the cancer diagnosis. These associations tend to survive the cancer care episode. That is true unless the patient blames that initial physician for overlooking early symptoms and delaying diagnosis and treatment—and that does happen. Many times a primary physician simply gets bypassed in a rush to specialized care for cancer.

When a retinue of specialists begins to parade into a case it often becomes a confusing matter to the patient. Specialists arrive on the scene in rapid succession without adequate introduction. Their role is not fully explained. Specialized diagnosticians and therapists appear in what, for the patient, feels like a hit-or-miss experience. Patient confusion and resentment adds burdens to the anxiety that already exists. Usually this occurs without either patient or physician realizing what is happening.

We discussed this a lot at Renewal. The most frequent feedback from group members to their peers in this situation was three things: First, organize your questions for the doctor and have them written down. Second, take a friend or relative with you to verify what you think you heard. Others suggest taking a tape recorder. And third, if you don't get what you need out of the present clinical relationship, find another doctor.

As a specialist who has dished out surgical opinions myself for many years, observing this phenomenon at our meetings made me appreciate more fully what haste and lack of preparation can do to a fragile relationship. Inconsistent or contradictory information causes bewilderment for patients on the receiving end. I learned from that, and when I saw one of my patients was angry, I began by asking, "Are you mad at me?" Sometimes that was the case. Usually it was something else. Maybe they were irritated that day about traffic or not finding a convenient parking spot. Maybe we kept them waiting too long. Maybe it was something in this avalanche of recent events that confirmed they were no longer in control. If I could identify the real issue there was a chance to move to a meaningful dialogue, not ritualize the conversation.

It is unusual to find a physician who does not have an opinion on virtually every subject, so that is not the problem. The greater the degree of specialization the more likely this is to be true. I know a gastroenterologist who starts every sentence with, "I think..." including social situations. After this start he often has to pause, realizing he hasn't formed an opinion yet about what is being discussed. He recovers quickly and says whatever pops into his mind next, appropriate or not. This projection of insecurity and arrogance only becomes important to us in the context of a clinical setting. Boorishness like this can be ignored but not if it comes from a physician you need to relate to. Hopefully their dynamic of diagnose ➤ treat can be separated by other important steps. It should be: *listen first* ➤ diagnose ➤ *listen* ➤ treat or prescribe ➤ *listen again.*

Jerome Groopman, MD, recently wrote an excellent book, *How Doctors Think* (Houghton Mifflin, 2007), that delves into this subject in a revealing way. How a doctor thinks is something most patients never consider. Really, how does my doctor think? One of the things Dr. Groopman concludes is that most medical errors (making a wrong diagnosis or choosing the wrong treatment) are due to flaws in physician thinking, not making technical mistakes. Another conclusion of his book is based upon research revealing that for a successful encounter, and for the patient to be persuaded to follow a doctor's advice, there needs to be both trust and a sense of mutual liking.

Dr. Groopman says other things I like. One, after finishing his manuscript he came to realize, "I can have another vital partner who helps improve my thinking, a partner who may, with a few pertinent and focused questions, protect me from the cascade of cognitive pitfalls that cause misguided care. That partner is present in the moment when flesh-and-blood decision-making occurs. That partner is my patient or her family member or friend who seeks to know what is in my mind, how I am thinking."

Someone else once said the only thing that matters in effective doctor-patient relationships is the physician having compassion and desire to help the patient, plus the patient having trust and confidence in the physician. Where the encounter takes place, the insurance coverage, the method of payment for services, none of that is very important.

Your physicians have plenty of information. Perhaps they are offering you the best opinion available anywhere. But if you perceive them in a negative way, knowledge may not be enough to carry your decision-making to a successful conclusion. Sometimes the physician's attitude is too rigid and precludes the patient from joining the decision. One woman in Renewal reported she had gone to see a surgeon well-recognized as a cancer expert. She told us this at her first meeting with the group. She was mad she had not known how to express her fear of a mastectomy. I knew the surgeon she went to see; he had been one of my mentors and I respected him a great deal. This woman explained to us she was searching for someone she could get to listen to her side of the story. She knew she had breast cancer; it already had been confirmed by a needle biopsy. Before she got to finish what she wanted to say this surgeon interrupted her. His manner was not rude, but he was firm, "Madam, knowing what I know, I cannot accept you as a patient unless you agree to have a mastectomy. It would not be ethical of me to treat you any other way." She came to us frustrated, and then went on to find someone else to be her surgeon.

—◠◠◠—

MARTIN was a man who came to Renewal at the urging of his daughter. He is an example of what happens in a relationship if your physician is moving too fast. Martin had come to stay with his daughter on the West Coast to continue convalescence. He already had definitive surgery for his cancer in Boston. Martin was a very successful Midwest businessman, a smoker, who had been diagnosed with lung cancer. He knew what he was looking for, he wanted the best. He took it upon himself to do some investigating of his own. He concluded the best surgeon in the entire country to remove the tumor practiced at a certain hospital in Boston. Once Martin had made this determination, arrangements were made by telephone. He flew to Boston, x-rays and all other test results in hand. He saw the surgeon in clinic the same day. Martin told us it was a brief visit but an agreement was made to proceed with what needed to be done. Martin was about sixty. He had been in the business world a long time, long enough to make his decisions quickly. "The surgeon seemed to be an OK guy," Martin told us.

When Martin made this first appearance at Renewal he was quite open. The brief version of his story was, that encounter in the clinic was about all Martin ever saw of his surgeon. Martin was admitted after the outpatient visit. A routine workup was completed by the house staff. A place on the surgery schedule had been reserved for the next day and everything moved ahead quickly. Martin said he had been disappointed that he was already asleep before the senior surgeon arrived. "At least I guess he showed up," he admitted with some uncertainty.

"Then after the operation it was three or four days before I saw my surgeon," Martin continued. "About five o'clock one afternoon he came and opened the door of my room. He didn't come in, just stood there with one hand holding his briefcase and the other still on the door handle." Martin paused like some thought had just occurred to him besides what he was saying, "He said everything was fine but he had to leave town to make a presentation at a surgical meeting. He was on his way to the airport. Said I would be discharged in a few days. Then he left—quickly. He was there 15, maybe 20 seconds."

A few days later a member of the resident staff came in and told Martin he was well enough to be discharged. "He told me I should get a hotel room and stay in town for a few more days in case I had any trouble, but that I'd be fine. Since I was from out of town I didn't have to come back." Martin started pulling the left side of his shirt out of his trousers, wanting to show the group an area of concern, then decided it wasn't necessary. He poked his shirt back into place. "I had the stub of a drainage tube still coming out between my ribs when I left. It had a little plastic bag stuck around it to catch the dripping. The resident said to just leave it until it fell out, and it did."

Martin actually did not have any complications. After all, he had a first rate surgical team. For Martin there just was something vaguely unsettling about the whole thing. But what? Now the surgery was over. Martin was on his own again. What was supposed to come next? After staying in the Boston hotel for a few days as he was told to do, Martin changed his mind about going home. Instead when he went to the airport he boarded a plane to Seattle to stay with his daughter. The daughter knew her dad. He had always been in control and made the decisions. Now he was in a position of not knowing what to do. She did the research, found Renewal, and convinced her dad to let her bring him to the meetings.

This is not going to become a right/wrong dynamic. Some things happen and we go on. In my role with Renewal I usually suggested a person go back and see their physician to resolve any problems. That wasn't practical in Martin's case. Go and state what the need is; say how you as patient see things. Say how you feel about the situation. If that doesn't work the first time, go back. I know a lot of people feel too intimidated to take a step like this. It's like the doctor can't be approached but that is wrong.

You'd really do your physician a favor by giving honest feedback. What is true in sales or the service industry is also true in practicing medicine: if you get a complaint take it seriously. For every person who expresses displeasure there are probably nine others who didn't bother—they just took their business somewhere else. If a physician is busy he or she may not notice. Our stories here are meant to help you understand your physicians and to get what you want from relationships with them.

Sir William Osler is one of those famous physicians everyone in medicine likes to quote. So I'll use him to tell you Sir William used to admonish students never to be satisfied with the ninety per cent of patients who express their appreciation. He said, in effect, go look for that other ten per cent. Find out why they didn't come back. They are the source of the wisdom you need to acquire.

How do patients get what they need, especially at critical times like deciding on therapy for cancer? You as patient may not get everything you want but you have to clarify what you really need. And, the perception of what you need may change as more is learned. You may be required to make an assessment about the skill, personality, and character of the physician taking care of you. You may need to decide whether choosing another physician or outside consultation is necessary.

Here's how you can visualize this relationship: Draw a straight line across a sheet of paper, like an arrow with a point at each end. Let this be the physician. Under one arrowhead list attributes of a person who projects warmth, converses freely. Someone who waits to talk after you have finished speaking. This physician also accepts multiple issues from you to deal with in a single visit. At the opposite end of your arrow, list words to describe a physician know-it-all. He or she is formal, maybe egotistical, pedantic, and interrupts you to give an opinion. He or she leaves the impression it's going to be my way or the highway. In the center of the line you have drawn put characteristics of someone who is friendly enough, but is running late, harried, pre-occupied, and may or may not have time to listen. He or she mostly wants to know "What's your main problem?" and "That's all we have time for today."

Now draw a second line under the first and put directional arrowheads on each end. Put personal characteristics for a patient here. At one end list what you think describes someone with little medical knowledge who is anxious, scared, uncertain, and confused. Maybe that person is forgetful, really doesn't grasp their own problem and needs lots of support and/or reassurance. Then go to the other end. Describe someone highly educated or experienced in medical matters. This person may be analytical, technical by nature, or naturally inquisitive. And in the middle of these two extremes put characteristics of someone open to facts, wanting to understand. This person is stable and just wants the straight story and honesty.

This is an aid for linking physician and a patient attributes together. As you align those two lists of characteristics you can see how some people will find a person similar to themselves in the exam room. There is a likelihood the two of them hit it off right away and have a meaningful conversation. If you as patient are at one extreme and the physician is a polar opposite, you may be dealing with someone who will not understand you. That person may be incapable of meeting your needs.

It is important to see that one is not right and the other wrong. This is about personality and preferences. A given medical professional and a given patient just may be different in their perceptions. A physician may give you good advice with a condescending attitude that causes you to feel insulted. On the other hand if you want facts and specifics and you have a kindly physician wanting to commiserate about your feelings, you too may leave the office without getting what you came for.

Someone has estimated that 85% of physicians are introverts. That is not bad (some of the extroverts in medicine are insufferable) but it does mean you may have to draw them out to understand their thinking. This has much to do with personal preferences and the mode in which physicians operate. Our thinking preferences, and we all have them, form the basis for why some people choose to go into medicine and once there, why they choose a certain field of specialization. This concept relating preferences to professions originates in the work of Ned Hermann and his brain dominance theory. Mansfield (Manny) Elkind of Mindtech, Inc., writes and lectures on this subject if you want to learn more.

The goal is to get what you want. Your physician should be the one making allowances for effective communication but that may not happen. If you find things are not going well, odd as it may seem, you the patient may be the better one to take control of the conversation. You may need to slow down a fast talker on the move. Ask for feedback after you speak to test whether you have been understood. Another strategy is to draw things out, asking that crucial issues be explained again. You may need to make a rapid adjustment and prioritize what can be accomplished in the short time allotted to a particular visit. It never hurts to inquire, "Do you have a few more minutes?" Ask questions. Take notes if you need to and say, "Now, did I get this right?" Request another appointment if necessary. Never lose your focus on getting the assistance you require.

— Bernie Siegel, MD —

As mentioned in the Introduction and several other places, Dr. Bernie Siegel was my inspiration in starting the Renewal group. He had done a similar thing a few years earlier with his Exceptional Cancer Patients (ECaP) which he described as that minority of people willing to try and do something for themselves. They did not just follow instructions blindly. More important to me was that he was a surgeon in a private practice group just like I was. This was not some government-sponsored and monitored initiative. It was not some university program dreamed up as a research project. As Bernie explained in his first book, *Love, Medicine and Miracles*, there were some people who seemed to confound conventional wisdom about their serious prognosis. Even more important, such people valued life enough to want to become proactive about getting well.

At a critical juncture in my life when I wanted to do more (and knew there was more) Bernie appeared. Without a lot of confirmatory evidence Bernie articulated his belief and then began to act upon it. The fact that practically no one else was doing what he did, or saying what he espoused, did not deter him. And just seeing one person do what Bernie was doing kept me from being deterred as well. I was even more impressed later. I found out that Bernie got a tremendous amount of mail and that he answered it personally...all of it! I saw some of that correspondence because some Renewal members wrote him. Even if there was just one sentence, scribbled as a response across the writer's own letter of inquiry, it came across as an honest and appropriate nudge of encouragement.

Years ago I was deeply affected hearing Bernie say to an audience, "We just need to decide if we want to go on..."

He was speaking about approaching obstacles in a more child-like manner. Realize what a child is like and what forms a child's impressions. We can read in the literature of child-rearing the opportunity we have to create positive impressions. With children it is important not to rebuke them with warnings of, "Don't!" Children only imprint images based upon what they experience. "Don't" makes no sense if there is no don't for a child to see; it's an abstraction.

Similarly, we adults have to choose whether we want to be "happy" or "right." Trying to be right all the time chains us in a very small room of existence. Where is the window? Where is the door? Seek forgiveness and release your self whenever necessary. Ask in person if you can. If that's not possible, write letters to whomever you need to contact. This works even if you write someone already dead. You missed your chance when they were alive—do it now. The value is for you. Unburden your self and arm the subconscious. We need to control our treatment when we are sick. Look for healers who are models to learn from. Their stories are written all over history. Like Bernie and others in this chapter, they exist now.

This probably sounds crass, but we need to learn how to use our doctors. Not everything your doctor was taught is currently correct. Information changes. And in our expectation of a towering medical intellect to advise us, remember that 50% of all doctors graduate in the lower half of their medical class. Be aware that some doctors may have been idealistic at one time in their development but may have succumbed now to a materialistic viewpoint. With cognitive care being paid proportionally less than in the past, some physicians have adopted an attitude that they are deserving. They feel they have a right to the trappings of success.

As suggested in a couple of places, you the patient may be in a position to help your doctor. For one thing recognize if you have a recurrence of your cancer, or if you are not responding to treatment, your physician may feel the same sense of defeat you do. We may have to pass through a moment where we are supporting our physician so he or she can support us. Can you heal the healer so that you too may be healed?

There is always an opportunity to approach your doctor in another way. Realize that when most physicians go to big medical meetings they have an expectation of being fawned over, being given trinkets and many other small gifts. This sounds foolish, but such do-dads are accepted as a sign of respect, of homage, even a sort of vindication when a physician feels beaten up by his or her employer or their practice. Accept this even if what I describe doesn't sound particularly healthy. Why do I tell you this? Because if that professional relationship isn't going well right now, I encourage you to try giving your doctor a "gift". Make it something small like a plant or something you have made. Deliver it and give your doctor a hug (but be prepared for anything the first time you try hugging—maybe you should ask!) and try to say a few words about how much you value the relationship. Tell your doctor about your experiences. Become a person in his or her eyes, not another diagnosis or "patient." As you advance in understanding your self, share what is working for you with your physician.

When I asked Bernie recently what he saw, looking back upon 30 years of working with people, speaking at workshops, communicating with so many thousands of people, he summarized it this way: First, so many things that were conjecture 30 years ago have become scientific mainstream. The healing power of humor has scientific validation, music therapy has broad application, and what we now know about the changes in our internal chemistry are but a few of the things that have found legitimacy.

Second, it is now credible to say that some people are able to renew themselves simply by going home to have fun. Bernie recently had an email from a man in London. The man had been given a hopeless prognosis for his cancer. Because of this he decided to sell everything, take his money and go have fun. Now he was doing so well that he suspects a mis-diagnosis. He had gotten rid of everything. "How do I get my medical records?" he asked, perhaps in jest. "I want to sue!"

People sometimes get better just by the simple expedient of enjoying life. This is connected to some extent to the Born Again movement. Cancer patients make what we must conclude are genetic, physical changes. It's the same as getting immunization shots and rebirthing themselves. These reborn people wind up with a new body. Even when it turns out they are rewarded with a five-year extension of life rather than their original two-year prognosis, that's an improvement.

Third, we can see now that survival behavior has common themes. What helps you get through everything you have to face? Talk to drug addicts and alcoholics that reclaim their lives. In AA they say, "Fake it until you can make it!" That can work for cancer too. We need to practice in our planning of next steps. We need to rehearse what we want and act it out until the time we finally meet with success.

Ask a United States Marine. He or she will tell you about their instruction: Do the right thing over the easy thing. Never give up! The Marine Corps also teaches, "Pain is just weakness leaving the body!" The Bible says, Gain your life by losing it. Live in the moment like all other animals do. When we pet a dog or other pet we release oxytocin. It makes us feel better. It's similar to the reason women tend to live longer than men. Women are more open and in touch. They form relationships men usually don't. For those of us trying to guide our patients and help people help themselves, realize that we can only coach. We can't do the change. "Go with your feelings, not your head," Bernie advised in closing. "If you find you only have 15 minutes to live, eat chocolate."

— O. Carl Simonton, MD —

About the same time I met Bernie I also met Dr. Carl Simonton. He started his career being a board-certified therapeutic radiologist. Then he began to have some experiences with his patients that changed the direction of his life. He and his coauthors wrote a number of papers related to their clinical findings. They also wrote a book, *Getting Well Again* (JP Tharcher, 1978). The book was a perennial favorite with the members of Renewal. It was a small book, but very concise in its message about patients taking charge of their illness. More recently Carl and a patient wrote another book, *The Healing Journey* (Authors Choice Press, 2002). For years he has been holding intensives in a small group setting at his facility in California.

At one time years ago Carl, as Bernie Siegel before him, came and spoke at a public forum for our community hospital. In both instances the Renewal group was the sponsoring organization. Both times the behind-the-scenes work was done by Renewal. That participation gave everyone involved a real sense of ownership to hear the philosophy our members adopted spoken about by such experts. These presentations were an affirmation of the very things we were trying to accomplish in our meetings.

Carl has continued to put on programs in California, but also now devotes most of his time to working abroad. Over the last 10-12 years Carl has refined standardized treatment and training models based upon data from his own work and the work of others in the field. He has found working in Germany, Japan, and now a center in Poland to be rewarding because the audiences are so receptive. With so much now being known about mind-body interactions he has been frustrated at how conventional medicine in the US has ignored, even opposed, so many practical findings.

The treatment models revolve around two major changes. The first is Carl's recognition of cognitive behavioral therapy, a discipline that he began to incorporate in 1987. The methodology for this is laid out in Carl's book, *The Healing Journey*, starting on page 69. Briefly he explains our problems begin with the beliefs and decisions we develop as a consequence of traumatic events in our lives. They can be something current like a diagnosis of cancer, or decades old, something that happened to us when we were younger. This type of therapy is a tool for addressing these unhealthy beliefs and moving away from them. Eastern cultures have had something similar, a process of thought transformation, for at least 2000 years—so this is not exactly new. It is incorporated in what the Dali Llama talks about as "the art of happiness."

217

The second major change in Carl's approach is an outgrowth of his attraction to Buddhist thought. This interest was helped along by a man he met in Germany whose work centers on translating Buddhist writings into other languages. He recommended the best works for Carl to read. A man named Thich Nhat Hanh has written several small books including *The Heart of Buddha's Teaching* that explain this in detail. The central Buddhist thought in this, which Carl was able to apply in a practical way, is conscious breathing. It is a simple ritual of breathing in, out, in, out in a slow, measured way. The attention is kept focused on the breathing process. Even six to eight repetitions of conscious breathing can have a beneficial effect. Carl has found this helps him personally in dealing with the exhaustion of international travel from going to his workshops (he does four in Germany and two in Japan each year). This technique deals with low energy and similar feelings. It is so simple that it is largely ignored or taken for granted. The basic technique does not require any complicated steps or deep study to be effective.

The week-long intensives are essentially the same whether conducted in the United States or abroad. In dealing with cancer patients and similar serious problems, Dr. Simonton tries to state clearly what the objectives are. The hope is that the attendee will develop tools to deal with the stresses in his or her own life—emotional and otherwise. Carl has come to believe that the number one stressor in everyone's life is in their primary relationship. It arises from the communication problems we have in cohabitation. At the beginning of the intensive goals are clearly stated. Even with such cautions it is important not to expect too much. Carl encourages the members of every group to be realistic. If there are expectations for the session that are too great, such as expectation of immediate cure, Carl tries to address that on the first day of the session.

When I asked Carl to reflect back on the thirty years he has been in this field, counseling primarily cancer patients, he started by saying, "The more I do this work, the more I see how it all flows and is interconnected." He related how a young woman had come up to him following a two-day workshop in Italy. She handed him a book she wanted Carl to read. He had never heard of either the book or its author. Protesting that he might not read it, he accepted the book. He did read it and was rewarded by finding it full of wisdom. The book is *Ultimate Healing* by Lama Zopa Rinpoche (Wisdom Publications, Somerville MA, 2001).

Stimulated by Carl's comments I got a copy of *Ultimate Healing* and read it too. In addition to chapters dealing with depression, purification, and healing meditations, the Editor's Preface contains several provocative assertions. Among them, Lama Zopa states he has found in his healing courses participants are often more interested in peace of mind than in curing their disease. The author goes on to say that "...disease itself has no external cause. In the West, however, the external conditions for a particular disease are usually regarded as its cause"—like bacteria and viruses. From his viewpoint, "Recovery from cancer and other diseases through meditation is now almost as common as recovery through standard medical treatment."

Carl then repeated the essence of three quotes that he feels are very important to understand if we plan to participate in our own healing process. The first looks back at the ancient history of medicine from Hippocrates. It essentially says, "Every person should know that from his brain, and only his brain, comes all his joy and all his suffering." Carl then quoted Sir William Osler, whom most physicians call the father of modern medicine: "Don't tell me what kind of disease the patient has; tell me what kind of person has the disease." The third quote is from Dr. Albert Schweitzer, probably the most widely known physician of the 20th Century. Carl related a story that the doctor told his nursing students training in Africa. (Once a woman physician in Germany, who formerly had been a nursing student with Dr. Schweitzer in Africa, rose in the audience at Carl's seminar to confirm that she had actually heard the famous doctor say this.) "Every person has within them this wise physician that best knows what they need to do to move in the direction of health..."

The most recent time Carl and I talked he mentioned another author and book, Eckhart Tolle's *A New Earth: Awakening Your Life's Purpose* that has impressed him very much. Guided by such wisdom and using the teaching techniques he has developed, Dr. Simonton works with his clients in small groups with the goal of showing them more joy and less suffering.

— Larry Dossey, MD —

A couple of years after I met Larry Dossey he published his first book, *Space, Time and Medicine* (1982). I separately knew about him because we had a friend in common, a surgeon in Dallas. Both Larry and my friend practiced at the same suburban hospital. Larry got interested in biofeedback as a treatment modality. He started an innovative biofeedback lab and that experience led to efforts to broaden its use in the medical community. Part of this effort grew out of self interest because Larry had his own troubles with migraine headaches. After this initial work he became interested in relaxation techniques and meditation. His experience in trying to conform to conventional practice expectations within a large multi-specialty group of internists, plus the time he devoted serving as Chief of Staff at his hospital, was too much. Larry retired from practice and moved to New Mexico. He has published at least nine other books. Starting with the publication of *Healing Words* (1993) his work chronicles an evolving appreciation of the value of prayer in healing.

One of the first things Larry wanted to express when he met with me in May, 2007, was his view that as time passes, the research on the value of prayer continues to become even more solid. When *Healing Words* was first published it was described as simply uncovering the enormous amount of evidence that already existed showing the effect prayer could have on the practice of medicine. In that book Dr. Dossey began to explain that the primary function of prayer is not to simply extend life or eradicate illness. Prayer helps sick people feel a connection to something beyond themselves. He feels this aspect deserves more emphasis than a simple judgment of whether people are cured or not. He says prayer is not some nifty new tool to be distributed to medical students and added to their bag of tricks. Another extension of this work is the concept Larry developed of the non-local mind. Non-local mind has become an emerging image helping explain what consciousness is all about. Many research studies require arcane methodology because of the nature of obtaining proof with scientific rigor.

Dr. Dossey emphasizes that spirituality is not synonymous with physical health. We must differentiate between our spiritual self and our physical self. Otherwise we impede our development with thoughts like, "Why did I get this illness?" Or, "Why was I born with this infirmity?" A man who is a champion cyclist can still get testicular cancer. A woman can be a fitness fanatic and still get breast cancer. A distance runner can still die from a heart attack. We have to accept this so we can come to terms with it.

There are even some negative aspects of spirituality that are important to understand. Pitfalls arise in trying to associate becoming ill with illness being something caused by sin. Illness is not some form of retribution. It is not caused by the devil. We are not being punished when we become ill. The question remains, what does an illness mean? So it does not become entangled in rituals from our past, one guide in mobilizing prayer is to simply hold to practical requests such as asking, "Let the best thing happen," and ending with, "Thy will be done."

— N. Michael Murphy, MD —

Dr. Murphy is another physician with a spiritual aspect to his work. He had a lot to do with my re-education on the subject and my own personal renewal. His parents were Irish as the name suggests even though he was born in the UK. His father and two brothers all joined the British Army in 1912 because conditions in Ireland offered few jobs. Michael went to medical school in Dublin then emigrated from there to America to study psychiatry. He also wanted to get away from his alcoholic mother. "But she came with me [he means figuratively] and it took years to let her go." While working in Albany, New York, he founded a hospice in 1977. He worked there for 17 years. "I left the hospice because it was being swallowed up by all the attention to the bottom line, and funding for staff training dried up. That was unacceptable to me," he told me.

The concept of caring for people in need is, of course, ages old, but what we know today as hospice, is actually a very recent concept. Hospice is a specialty caring for people in the last stage of life. It is something that we've touched upon several times in this book, because dying is inextricably linked to living whether we wish it to be that way or not. Many people in society can choose to ignore this truism, but most people with serious diseases like cancer cannot. We first envisioned a free-standing hospice in our community in the late 1980s. This gave Gerri Haynes and me a chance to work together, recruiting experts from around the world to come and advise us in our planning. One of those experts was Dr. Murphy.

Michael stayed with my family on our farm a number of times when making these consulting trips to the Northwest. He and I quickly became friends. Over the years we began to consider each other as brothers and even to identify ourselves publicly as such. Michael had relatives in Vancouver, Canada, and would generally stop to visit us when he went to visit them in addition to his consulting work for the hospice. During this same period he developed workshops, first on Death and Dying for those interested in hospice, and later on Love, Loss, and Forgiveness for the general public. He finally moved to Ireland in 2004 to re-discover his roots in the south of that country and, as he says, to bring his father's soul and spirit home.

Here is one of the many observations Dr. Murphy shared with me in our private correspondence. He quoted from Anatole Broyard something thought-provoking for me and possibly of use to you: *"A doctor's job would be so much more interesting and satisfying if he would occasionally let himself plunge into the patient, if he could lose his fear of falling…the mood of the hospital might have to be modified. It might be less like a laboratory and more like a theater…he must see that his silence of neutrality is unnatural…In learning to talk to his patients, the doctor may talk himself back into loving his work."*

Michael met with the Renewal group on several occasions. These were always rousing, free-wheeling sessions that we all loved. Mike told stories with warmth, patience, humor. His message in those stories made for some great meetings. He brought the perspective of both a wise physician and an experienced psychiatrist. As far as I know he developed the concept of the Family Meeting around serious illness. This became a prelude to death with emancipation through forgiveness. Such preparation obviously has implications for how we live, not just how we prepare to die. Michael is someone experienced by countless dealings with dying hospice patients and their families. He has some unconventional insights into what is lacking in hospice and the practice of American medicine in general, something we are trying to reveal in this chapter. And, with this short introduction, Michael has several topics and can speak for himself.

—⁂—

Family Meetings: I started family meetings early on in the life of our new hospice in Albany. The idea was based on my training in psychiatry related to family dynamics. We invited the whole family to attend—including small children. What I did was influenced by the fact that I was not present at my own mother's death. I never had the opportunity at that time to say in words what I needed to say. The fact is that had I been present, I would more than likely have been speechless. There would have been nobody there to guide me; I would not have had the courage to speak about how difficult her alcoholism was for me, how difficult it was to have been her child with all her clinging and seductiveness.

In the early days of family meetings, I acted the psychiatrist, distancing myself from the family. I was there interpreting unnecessarily, and failing to address the elephants in the room. It was only after introducing training for the staff and participating in experiential workshops that I became more lovingly compassionate. I became a more helpful guide to the dying and to their families. In the training, when we imagined that we were dying and only had ten minutes to speak to the important people in our lives before we died, I was able at last to speak to my mother.

In just a couple of minutes I was able to say something like, "Mom, being your son was very difficult for me. When I was small, you were so demanding of my love because Dad had no idea how to love himself or anyone else. I was uncomfortable being with you and even more uncomfortable being away at school. Then your alcoholism created such a barrier between us and I felt angry and helpless, so I eventually ran away to America. But you are my Mom, and you gave me many gifts—humor and imagination being not the least of them. I want to thank you for being my Mom. Forgive me for running away in one way or another. I would like to bless you and receive a blessing from you."

That is what I would have liked to have said. Amazingly, saying it long after she was dead still allowed me to become much more peaceful with the mother within. And, maybe she heard! No confrontation, and no blame, just a loving touch. Perhaps I thought I wanted to know why she was such a weird mother or why she drank. I know she did not know the answer to that. Blame-filled questions like that are unskillful and useless. They are not what we really want to say. We are dying to say, "We missed out on one another quite a lot. I love you. Please forgive me, and I forgive you. Thank you so much for bringing me into this world. Let's bless one another!"

So the family meetings entered a new phase after about 10 years. They became more lovingly effective in making peace and saying goodbye. After I left the hospice, one social worker continued family meetings and still does, but the leadership no longer gives it the priority it had in the past. The frequency of such meetings now is rare. In general professionals say that if the family asks, they would do a family meeting. Most families will not ask. They say they don't need one or that they already are very close. My experience is that every family needs a family meeting as a routine. It especially should be encouraged for all who enter the hospice as staff, patients or families.

Doctor and Nurse Training in Death and Dying (and in Living): Doctors and nurses are not prepared. They are taught never to say die, and they are also not prepared for their own death, or the deaths of their loved ones, nor their patients. This lack of preparation has not improved much over the years despite some training in death and dying. That's because the training is neither experiential nor built into graduate and postgraduate training from beginning to end. Physicians and nurses need to be guided to imagine their own death and the deaths of their loved ones in experiential training. They need to practice saying what they have to say and not just imagine dying theoretically if they are to become able to be fully present for dying patients and their families. So doctors and nurses *all* need a family meeting if they are to be holistically prepared. Medicine and nursing are arts as well as science, and dying is as much a subject for healing as is living.

Lack of training in both living and dying causes burnout in professional caregivers. Failure to take care of their own needs and their own self-esteem and loving nature causes caregivers to run out of compassion. If we love and have compassion for ourselves, we will never exhaust healing energy. I have seen over the years some awful dying and deaths, among physicians in particular. I have seen very many practicing physicians angry at the system and everyone around them because they failed to give themselves loving care. They don't know how to do it. Continuing education never encourages them to spend at least half their Continuing Medical Education in self-care. For the past 15 years I have devoted myself to developing and facilitating workshops on *Love, Loss & Forgiveness* for health care professionals and others. These have been very successful in Europe where there is more receptivity for this training and recognition of the need. Professionals in the US will usually devote no time to this "soft" experiential training, and would sooner have heart attacks than risk the more treatable and creative heart breaks.

Hospice Care in the Twenty-first Century: Like in every other field of "scientific" endeavor, hospices have been taken over by big business and big medicine. Hospices have lost some or much of the loving and caring touch just as obstetrics was diminished in the takeover by "masculine medicine." The "medicalization" of hospices in the US has meant that the bottom line is first priority. More and more technical and pharmacological treatments are used at the expense of the Family Meeting that took place with *every* family in the earlier days of our hospice. Hospice staffs are often the warmest of people, but failure to provide them with the self-training they need has led to a decline of doing what needs to be done. Most people who are dying are unable or unwilling to approach the healing that is possible at the end of life, or at any other time, without being encouraged to do so. If staff is unprepared or unaware of the possibilities, then this opportunity for healing is missed. Unfinished business will be handed down for succeeding generations to contend with.

With cancer or anything else, we will not survive well and we will not heal if we fail to love ourselves. The good news is that learning to love ourselves is possible at any stage in life. Hospices in general and medicine in particular have very limited understanding of the power and place of love in healing. Love in the US is generally thought of as "unprofessional" and dangerous, since love and sex are usually thought of in the same manner. Hospitals may provide a place in which humans can be fixed, and hospices may provide a place in which they may die, but without love there will be little warmth and healing for staff, patients, or families.

A Few Thoughts about Forgiveness: The idea of forgiveness was co-opted by the established churches, and involved forgiving others who trespassed against us and vice versa, and also asking God to forgive us our sins. These notions are very distracting from the down-to-earth approach to forgiveness that we need to take. We cause ourselves endless unrest and suffering by holding onto stories of betrayal, abuse, and other hurts. Forgiveness is letting go of those stories so that we will no longer suffer on their account. Unconditional love of self or others is impossible when we are weighed down with past pain, and we need to let go.

In my workshops on *Love, Loss & Forgiveness*, participants have the opportunity to "speak to" those who have caused pain and suffering. They also speak to those whom they have betrayed, abused, or hurt, including themselves. We are able to do that because the one we need to speak to is the one we hold captive inside ourselves, and not the one (alive or dead) who has hurt us. It is the mirror image of that person we have allowed inside. It is the same one who may have plagued us day and night for endless years. We need to speak to that image. We speak not in a raging, judgmental, argumentative manner, but by saying that we need to let go of the story and say goodbye to it because it is killing our spirit and our soul. We might even say that it is sad that we were not able to make our relationship more fruitful, but there it is. "I wish you well, and may you be in peace," is the thing to say. That is all we need to do! We may need to repeat it a few of times, but it works!

— Walter M. Bortz II, MD —

Without straying too far from our theme about Renewal and cancer, I want you to at least know about Dr. Walter Bortz. He is still a practicing internist and geriatrician. He is an accomplished speaker—I might say a fearless speaker—whom I have known for years and from whom I have learned a great deal. At the time of this writing Walter tells me he is 78 years old. He has been running marathons for 38 years and still runs several miles every day. (His beloved wife, Ruth Anne, outdid him for years by running ultra marathons in the range of 50 miles.)

Dr. Bortz usually writes or speaks on some aspect of the aging process. He has just finished his fifth book and written over 100 articles on health-related subjects. Some of the recurring themes are "Dare to be 100" and "Use It or Lose It". He was early in defining the problems of aging, is forceful in making his presentation to physicians, and is downright inspiring. Here are some ideas he shares with his audiences and in his writing:

Most of us reach our physical high point when we are about 20-25 years old. The weight you had then is usually your ideal weight. Most of us start gaining about a pound or two a year after that. Such an accumulated gain leads to a host of consequences, all of them bad. By about age thirty the average person begins their slow decline in physiological processes. That continues, on average, for another forty to fifty years. Ideally, with proper attention to diet and especially exercise, we can maintain most all of our organ function and physical capability during our adult working years. With organ function we're speaking principally about the heart, kidneys, and lungs.

We arrive at retirement still operationally intact. Even if we are not so good, with a moderate amount of attention to our health, we have declined at a functional rate of half of a per cent (0.5%) per year. Eighty or eighty-five per cent in old age is good (0.5% per year times 30-40 years). A graph of our organ reserve and physical capability through adult life plots out on almost a horizontal line. Inevitably a terminal event happens and we are going to die. Hopefully it is a sudden event or at least an abrupt downward turn in our life's course. We die without lingering or having time to suffer.

One of the troubles we have as a society is that either due to chronic disease, smoking, gaining weight, alcohol, or any number of other bad things we do to ourselves, we cause acceleration in the decline in our organ function. We decline faster than half a per cent a year. A one per cent yearly decline will still turn out to be acceptable. We still can retire with seventy or sixty per cent of function and live normally (1% times 30-40 years). With increasing misuse or disuse the rate of decline accelerates to two per cent rate each year. Multiply that rate by even thirty five years, we have set the stage for trouble just when we start collecting our Social Security checks.

As a generalization, most of our organs (again, our kidneys, lungs, heart), can keep us comfortable and ambulatory with a quarter of their original capacity remaining. It's just like living with only one kidney or one healthy lung; we do just fine. With two% decline we won't have much reserve left to deal with the stress of sudden emergencies like getting out of a burning house, a car wreck, or major surgery. We won't have reserves to make our remaining years of decline as comfortable as they might have been. Infection or injury can suddenly take us to the edge. As a generalization, once we drop below 20% remaining function, we will be restricted. We have no reserves. We become borderline and have set the stage for the frustration of incapacity in whatever time we have left. We develop a familiarity with the medical community we otherwise might have avoided.

We enter the realm of conventional medicine practice. Physicians do what they can to squeeze water out with diuretics. Medication makes the heart pump a little harder, maybe aided by a pacemaker. You get oxygen blown into your lungs through a nasal cannula while you carry a little green bottle everywhere you go. Walter's point is these functional challenges have become medical diagnoses. So many of these problems now requiring treatment were, for the most part, preventable.

I once heard Walter tell a disarming story to a large group of physicians in San Francisco. It was about his determination to wage a personal war against aging. He used humor, which is probably the best way to get through to a sophisticated audience of your medical peers. Physicians in such audiences are about as complacent and hard to change as their patients. Physicians also have an inherent conflict in listening to a talk about exercise and diet because treatment is their stock and trade, not prevention. No illness to treat and monitor equals no job. Besides, many physicians rationalize they already know how few patients listen to admonishments about lifestyle changes. Why bother? The truly knowledgeable in a given patient population, the devotees of good health, already know. They will not be coming in for office visits in the first place.

In a recently published article, Walter extended an open invitation to his 100th birthday — in 2030! In the same article he reiterated that believing you can live to 100 is the most important step. Walter constantly monitors reports on centenarians looking for factors that actually extended useful life. He concludes that most changes we see with aging are not aging per se but disuse, and thus preventable.

Another reason I think so much of Walter is the way he used to speak about his mother. When I first met him Walter regularly, and unabashedly, recounted conversations the two of them had and the pithy reflections his mother made on life. She was getting up in years and lived a few miles away from Walter's practice in Palo Alto. He visited her every day just like he took his daily run. She finally died peacefully in 1999 at age 95. He was proud to say, "She died at home. When she died she had no pain, she had no loneliness, she had no tubes. She was not taking any pills and, she had no diagnoses!"

As a final note, when I interviewed Walter by telephone for this book he was busy at his desk editing a book manuscript based upon recent observations in practice. He was full of frustration over this new subject. He was working to characterize the disaster that looms from 200 million Americans being at risk for diabetes. "We have gotten fat, and lazy," he told me, "who owns your health? Is it going to be owned by an institution like Kaiser? [Speaking of his California market.] It should be owned by you!" He writes his three central strategies are to have health replace disease as medicine's primary mission, have the practitioner replaced by the person as the primary agent of well being, and change financial incentives to being well, not being sick.

He now is ready to say that our most important organ is our wallet. Politics is strangling initiative and smothering solutions. As health care has become hopelessly politicized, we must find a new solution. He is ready to give up disease management as an operational failure. We need to incentivize health with the public, down at the individual citizen level. We need to undertake the stern task of making everyone personally responsible for caring for themselves. The new book fuses disease medicine with health medicine into what he calls "the next medicine." *Next Medicine* is out in 2009.

— David Sobel, MD —

Some notable work has been published by Dr. David Sobel with the Kaiser system in California. I did not know of his work when I started, but I later learned that Dr. Sobel has observed how effective patients can be in supporting and educating one another. This is especially true if the sharing can be compartmentalized into some specific field like diabetes, chronic lung disease, arthritis, or cancer (among others). More controversially he suggests extending the concept of a mature person, usually a woman or nurse in a community or neighborhood that becomes recognized as the local "go-to" person for practical advice. I mention this partly because this concept validated the experience of Renewal. On a larger scale this concept could be a way of doing good while at the same time recognizing the manpower problem of how to organize groups such as ours.

Medical economics is beyond the scope of this book, but Dr. Sobel speculated early on that perhaps only 15% of health problems are ever elevated to the level of seeking medical advice in the first place. Based upon this observation, fully 85% of what happens in a community, such as bouts of gastroenteritis, cuts and scrapes, fevers, the flu, pulled muscles and backaches, people either self-prescribe or ask a friend what they should do. Health care keeps requiring more from our economy each year (currently 16% of GDP and heading for 20%). Dr. Sobel points out that increasing the 85% who can take care of themselves with local support a few percentage points to 90% releases a huge amount of money and manpower to care for those who really need expert professional care. These funds could be shifted to preventive care for those who are uninsured or have no access. The basis for getting this to happen is support groups and mutual education. This would ameliorate our health care crisis and is a very attractive idea.

— Alastair Cunningham, Ph.D. —

During my investigations for information Renewal could use I came upon a program called The Healing Journey and its founder, Dr. Alastair Cunningham.

Although I do not know Dr. Cunningham personally, his work and his program are so significant I felt the reader needs to be aware of what he has accomplished. Dr. Cunningham and The Healing Journey are in Toronto, Canada, at Princess Margaret Hospital. Through his very informative website, the books and workbooks he has published, plus the onsite programs, there is much available to anyone with cancer.

When I contacted Dr. Cunningham during the preparation of this book he provided background information that makes an interesting story. Alastair was born in New Zealand and spent his early years there. He moved to Australia and received his Ph.D. in microbiology (cell biology) from the University of Canberra in 1967. He went back to New Zealand, and then spent several years in the U.S., England, then back to Australia, combining work, fellowships, and research. This was during the 1970s and consisted of basic research in immunology, investigating how the diversity of antibodies is generated. He wrote a textbook based upon his work, *Understanding Immunology*.

He eventually moved to Canada where he became Senior Scientist at the Ontario Cancer Institute/Princess Margaret Hospital. For most of this time he had an additional position as Professor of Medical Biophysics at the University of Toronto (1980-2005). He received a number of awards in recognition of his efforts.

He was drawn to immunology thinking this was the field that held the possible cure for cancers. In the usual connotation, that has not proven to be the case. He felt his immunology work wasn't doing any good and wanted to move to a field of investigation that had more practicality. He was looking for something that would have value to people. He became interested in mind/body interactions through study of psychology and yoga. While still doing immunology Dr. Cunningham began to change the direction of his investigation. He started doing experiments on conditioning responses in mice. He moved gradually into group support and training in coping skills for use by cancer patients, including benefits to patient quality of life. Since 1982 he has continuously been conducting such groups for cancer patients.

Dr. Cunningham took a sabbatical and went back to school to get a second Ph.D. in clinical psychology (1987). He helped establish the Well-spring Centre for Cancer Patients in Toronto, a program that now has spread all over Canada. In 1992 he published *The Healing Journey*, a book explaining to cancer patients what can be done to help oneself against this disease. In addition to a second edition of that book he also wrote *Bringing Spirituality into Your Healing Journey* (2002).

Years ago I first heard of *The Healing Journey* without connecting its work with Dr. Cunningham. At the time his program was described as having three parts:

Phase I - Taking control and how we react to our environment

Phase II - Getting connected and appreciating the value of under-standing ourselves

Phase III - Our search for meaning, realizing we are connected, not separate.

The program has evolved and become much more sophisticated. There are four levels to the program plus a "graduate" program. These are multi-week, onsite intensives that begin with lectures and focus on strategies and teach techniques. The real therapy is learning about one's own self. Attendees are given workbooks and have homework. Both books and workbooks can be ordered from the website. Levels 3 and 4 transition to become more interactive with group psychotherapy. Spouses may attend but have their own separate sessions.

In the preface to his book, *Can the Mind Heal Cancer?* (2005) Dr. Cunningham identifies himself as someone who had a serious cancer, Stage III colon cancer, in 1987. He talks about how he put his hypotheses to the test. He credits Lydia Temoshok with a theory about cancer that he briefly outlines: "[I]f we place undue stress or strain upon ourselves from an early age, we will be susceptible to later disease…And conversely, if we strive to undo these distortions, to reclaim our authentic selves when afflicted by cancer, we allow our innate healing mechanisms the best opportunity to overcome, or at least retard, the disease…We can say quite definitely that when people with cancer become involved in helping themselves psycho-logically and spiritually, they almost always enjoy a much better quality of life. It is highly probable, if not yet proven to the satisfaction of all, that some will live much longer as a result."

Dr. Cunningham goes on to identify the mental qualities people de-velop in their struggle with medically incurable cancers. His research indi-cates that the ones who greatly outlive their prognoses have these qualities: *autonomy*, or achieving a sense of free choice to live life as desired; which is related to *authenticity*, or learning one's true identity through introspective psychological and spiritual work; and *acceptance*, an attitude of tolerance, forgiveness, and ultimately love for other people, themselves, and all living things. He ends this description by saying, "It is perhaps not surprising that such a healed mental state promotes physical healing."

Dr. Cunningham feels the power of the Healing Journey program comes from the participants themselves. He feels that quality of life is improved by the programs and that their successive levels of sophistication are very rewarding to many—he just feels it is important not to create any dependency. Research continues finding out what objectively can be done at the psychological level to help cancer patients. Three randomized trials have shown that teaching practical coping skills (relaxation, mental imaging, thought monitoring) produce better results than support alone.

Another of his randomized, controlled studies using women with metastatic breast cancer failed to show any average effect of the intervention in prolonging life. Studies done elsewhere, usually with the same kind of patient population, also have failed to show prolongation of life. Dr. Cunningham feels positive effect definitely is there but concludes the very modest changes undertaken in most studies are not enough to demonstrate effect. Also, comparing group trials and lumping everyone together in meta-analyses obscures the effects of adjunctive psychological therapy. He believes more attention needs to be paid to the individual undergoing the therapy. He feels we are being arrogant when we devise a program where everyone gets the same treatment. The psychological realm is one place where treatment must be individualized to the patients' needs.

Many in the scientific community have concluded the mind cannot affect cancer. Dr. Cunningham reaches a different conclusion. He feels that what most studies have shown so far is that general supportive therapy, which is neither intensive nor designed to induce significant mental change, will not produce an average life-prolonging effect that is statistically significant. More than that in his opinion such programs would be like giving AIDS patients aspirin, then concluding that drugs won't affect the course of AIDS. Or, to make the analogy even more apt, it's like giving aspirin to AIDS sufferers and drawing conclusions when you know that many of those people don't take their medication (just like most people with cancer, and even many in support groups, make little use of what is offered).

Dr. Cunningham concluded our conversation with this statement: "I feel strongly that we risk making a mistake here that could deny many people the chance to live longer with cancer. Agreed, the evidence for prolongation of life by psychological therapy is slight as yet, but we simply have not done more than scratch the surface with our investigations. My clinical observations, as well as research over 30 years, have convinced me that at least some people with serious cancer can enjoy longer, as well as better quality, lives when they become involved with self-healing methods."

---——— CHAPTER 9
EXPLORING ILLNESS WITH A PHYSICIAN ———

"Be thankful for these moments of pain, for in pain
the mind is humbled...pain and illness would not serve
their purpose if they were not felt."
— *Param Sant Jaimal Singh Ji*

It has always seemed to me that a physician has an advantaged position to gain insight when he or she becomes seriously ill. In Chapter 6 I gave some personal examples. In my career as a surgeon there have been thousands of episodes that immersed me for a time in some person's life. Most of those washed by so quickly that I did not get a chance to learn from them. I got better at capturing the experience as years passed.

One instance involved a local gastroenterologist. I knew him as a member of our medical community for some twenty years. He was a native of South America and educated in England before coming to the Northwestern US to open his practice. He was witty, urbane, and always cheerful. As I learned after the fact, he had decided privately, and rather quickly, to turn his practice over to his associate and retire. He came in the office to see a few patients and said his goodbyes one Friday. That night he and his wife took his associate and her husband out for a celebratory dinner. My friend was in fine spirits. On Saturday morning he awoke with a headache. A short time later he collapsed and was taken to our hospital's emergency room. Tests revealed he had a large brain tumor. In another twenty-four hours he was dead.

He went from seeing patients on Friday to being dead on Sunday. This certainly is not a unique circumstance but it was a shock. It led to a good deal of introspection and self-consciousness, both of which were revealed a few days later at his memorial service. At the reception which followed, most of our colleagues circled into small groups. They spoke in cautious voices about the suddenness of it all. Sudden death like that leaves us shifting about in our private thoughts and speculation.

Unlike this instance, what we are going to do now is look at what happened to three physicians in our local community. None of them has been whisked away without warning. They are all still in practice and I have known them each for about 30 years. I have picked them as a way of letting you see illness from another side, the side of the physician. The first two had cancer. The third is a partner in my old surgical practice.

— HANS DANKERS M.D. —

Dr. Hans Dankers is a primary care physician I came to know when he joined a Family Practice group in a nearby small town. He and I had a professional association around referrals he would make to me as a general surgeon. I have known Dr. Dankers so long it seems natural to refer to him by his first name, Hans. He lived on a farm with his wife and two sons, raising sheep as an important family activity. He had been in practice for ten years when he developed a brain tumor. His surgery happened rather quickly but afterwards, during his convalescence, I had a chance to check on his progress. This was in 1990. By that time the Renewal group had been in existence for almost a decade. Hans attended our meetings for a time where he told his story just like everyone else and shared some of his insights.

It was apparent to me that many physicians could benefit from a better understanding of the personal effects of severe illness, especially hearing it from one of their peers. A few months later I arranged for Dr. Dankers to speak at one of our weekly hospital staff meetings. He related his experience quite effectively. His talk was even more effective because he was not fully recovered at the time. I still remember a neurologist in the audience being fascinated to hear Hans talk about the pain of having a cerebral angiogram. The neurologist, who must have ordered at least a thousand angiograms on patients, wanted Hans to tell him just what it had felt like. It was as if he felt this physician speaker was specially qualified to relate the details of the experience. It was obvious the neurologist at that moment was awakening to a thought about the discomfort part. It was all news to him—and certainly he never asked one of his patients about it.

Hans resumed his practice and still continues to see patients some eighteen years later. We don't see much of each other since I stopped practicing, but recently I paid him a visit at his home. Sitting by a wood fire with his white-muzzled Labrador retriever snoozing at his feet, he and I relived his experience.

Hans recalled he knew something major was wrong. For about three months he noted brief but increasingly frequent episodes of incoordination in his right hand (he is right-handed). He couldn't focus mentally... generally felt "off." He remembers the anxiety of not having any life insurance when he began to anticipate seeking medical advice. Up to that point he felt life insurance was something a young man like himself didn't need. A phone call to the local neurologist confirmed this was likely partial seizure activity. Hans scheduled his own appointment for an MRI. This test appointment was for late in the afternoon, 6:30 pm. Hans remembers how unfortunate that timing was because it came following an afternoon of festivities for his practice. That was the very day they held an open house for their new clinic facility. Hans told his wife Martha of his seizure activity as they drove together to get the MRI.

The MRI test showed a large tumor of three centimeters in the left premotor area of the brain. The local neurosurgeon saw him the next day. He in turn referred Hans to the University of Washington for brain mapping. Hans remembers this new neurosurgeon he met at University Hospital as being very kind. At the time of surgery, which was on March 17, the tumor proved to be a malignancy as expected. It was an astrocytoma, but one of the more favorable Grade I type and it had a low mitotic index. The surgical margins were mostly clear as revealed by the mapping technique, but as this tumor has indistinct borders, some of it had to be left on its deepest margin next to the ventricle. Because of the remaining tumor, a course of radiation therapy followed the surgery. This combined approach was successful. After all these years there has never been any recurrence.

Hans was aided in remembering these events because he kept a journal. Even from the first postoperative day he showed me his scrawling and rambling notations. They are recorded in a black, hardbound notebook he referred to during our conversation. He recalls numbness in his right hand when he woke up, opposite the side of the tumor, in the area innervated by the cancerous region of the brain. A more distressing consequence was that the areas controlling speech and cognition were involved. When the neurosurgeon first quizzed Hans with a question testing for medical knowledge, he asked, "How would you treat a urinary tract infection?" Hans remembers thirty seconds elapsing while he formulated an answer. He knew what he wanted to say but all he could articulate was, *"E. coli."* In other words, his answer gave a cause, not treatment.

He also recalls the postoperative hospital stay of five days being very difficult. Part of this was the frustration of losing control over events during his convalescence. When his arterial line was removed, Hans was sitting in a chair. He reacted with a moment of fainting. The nurse in attendance interpreted this slumping forward as evidence of a seizure. She insisted that her physician patient take additional Dilantin in the form of pills she hurriedly brought to the bedside. Hans knew he hadn't had a seizure and knew he already had too much Dilantin since he felt both bloating and nausea. He did not like the anti-seizure medications, which also included Decadron, because he felt they were contributing to his being constipated. Unable to verbalize what just had happened he clamped his teeth together in resistance. He resisted the medication but ultimately lost this contest of wills. The nurse was insistent and he had to do as he was told and swallow his medicine.

The recovery story is a lesson both in disease and treatment, linked with protracted consequences of what sometimes must be done. Early on Hans could read out loud and recite the Lord's Prayer. He could also say, "Now is the time for all good men to come to the aid of their country." He could not answer questions directly or turn a new thought into speech. The hardest thing he recalls is the effect on his wife and their two sons, ages eleven and nine at the time. His wife is a registered nurse and very involved in community activities. She is a wise woman. Hans remembers she not only was supportive during this convalescence, but conveyed her assumption that her husband would be OK. For the boys it was more difficult. This was about the time of the death of Sammy Davis, Jr. Because this was a prominent news item, the boys made an association and wanted to hear more assurance from their father. Hans found he could read to the boys, but spontaneous speech or conversation was very slow in returning.

While convalescing at home Hans tried to catch up on journal reading for continuing medical education credit. He understood what he was reading on these occasions, but at the end couldn't put the individual pieces of information together. He felt at least he could do things like organize the messiness in the family garage. Some tasks he could do. He especially remembers a frustrating incident when he looked at the tangled garden hose. He knew what the desired outcome of re-coiling the hose should look like. Despite a prolonged attempt he could not figure out how to accomplish what he wanted. Another time he took something apart to repair it, removing a set of screws. When it was time for reassembly, he could not figure out what he had done with the screws. He became very agitated at his own incompetence but just then his neighbor from next door stopped by and found the screws for him.

Six weeks after surgery Hans started back seeing patients. The attempt to resume his previous multitasking routine proved to be both frustrating and exhausting. It took twice as long to do the necessary charting. He had to take several additional weeks off. On the good side, he remembers his colleagues, the office staff, and his regular patients all being very kind and understanding. They were not the problem. It was when Hans went from patient to patient, tried to make treatment and administrative decisions, answer multiple phone calls with his halting speaking voice, plus all the outside activities like coaching a youth soccer team for his son, he realized he could not keep it all straight. He recalls a period of not sleeping well. He counted for the first time a total of thirteen trains passing by his house each night. He would awaken many mornings wishing the coming day was already over. He accepts now that he was depressed. He remembers his brain being in overdrive with too many thoughts about what might happen next.

As time passed the missing skills began to return and Hans was able to return to the clinic again. Despite the many frustrations, Hans's intellect was intact. As I questioned him Hans remarked he always has been compassionate. He has always been a giving person, supported causes, and been active in his church. He felt no radical departure from old ways was necessary. He did experience becoming more sensitive to anything he saw his patients having to go through. One of the first patients to come in after surgery was a person who had been seeing him for several years, a woman who had a right-sided stroke and could not speak. Another outgrowth of this heightened sensitivity was that others recognized it and realized the value of Hans's perspective. His partners began asking him to counsel people with similar problems from their own practices.

One of the first people to ask for help was the neurosurgeon who did his brain surgery. He asked Hans to return to the University Hospital and counsel another physician, a resident of Oregon, who had just undergone the same operation for a brain tumor.

When Hans walked back onto the neurosurgical ward at University Hospital it evoked a very negative emotion. The same nurse who had forced him to take the Dilantin pills happened to be on duty and he saw her. The noises on the daytime ward were particularly bothersome, such as the PA system announcements, the clanging of equipment—everything. Despite this reaction to old surroundings Hans proceeded to the private room of this other physician from Oregon and made an immediate connection with him. This other physician was still in bed. A large bandage was twisted around his head.

After a while their visit became almost intolerable to Hans because of distracting hospital noises outside the room. He got up, took some towels from the bathroom and stuffed them under the closed door. Finally he had to stuff pieces of tissue in his ears to block out the sounds even as their conversation continued. Being on the ward carried such an unpleasant association from his own recent hospitalization that Hans could barely remain to finish the visit.

Hans had thought his personal experience made him a good resource for talking to patients about cancer but this often was difficult. One instance he remembers is a man in Renewal [Gary] who had been operated upon for an advanced melanoma. Seeing him depressed Hans. It was difficult to give advice to someone who had such a poor prognosis.

The only outside event Hans associates with the course of his illness is the stressful effect of a prolonged malpractice suit. He delivered a baby in 1981. At four months of age the child suffered brain damage after having meningitis. The suit was not actually filed for another three years, but the allegation was out there. The suit alleged that failure to diagnose the child's meningitis during an initial twelve hours of symptoms was the cause of the damage and was Hans's fault. The suit took over two years to work its way through the courts. The verdict came back in Hans's favor—the jury found that he was not at fault. Still, this was something to live with for five years. For most doctors who are sued the psychological damage proves to be indistinguishably bad whether you are found liable or exonerated. Even now, after all these years, the pain of this experience is very near the surface.

Another event that has weighed heavily on Hans after his brain tumor is the unusual coincidence that his older sister also developed a brain malignancy. The sister's tumor was picked up on MRI because she had multiple sclerosis. The tests were being done on a serial basis to follow the progression of that disease. Her doctor noted something new that was different from the multiple sclerosis. It turned out to be a cancer on the right side of her brain. The sister had her surgery in 1993, just a couple of years after her brother and while he was still in his recovery phase. Because of the risk that postoperative radiation might potentiate the MS, she had surgery without additional treatment. She had a recurrence in 2003.

This was difficult for Hans to talk about. His sister started on chemotherapy and tried several innovative alternative therapies. Ultimately she developed two additional brain tumors which were biopsied and proved to be a high-grade, even more serious type of malignancy. She grew progressively weaker due in part to the aggressive treatment. Hans felt especially close to his sister because of the similarity in the paths of their cancers. He flew to visit her on a regular basis up until the time she died in 2006.

As time has passed, Hans is more philosophical about his illness and the consequences that followed treatment. He explained his own analogy of grief being like an escalator: It moves up and you can start stepping upwards to shorten the transition time, or you can just stand still. You can even walk backward if you want and prolong the time it will take you to get up to the next level. But no matter which choice you make about this, there will be levels of experience you will have to pass through, or endure. For Hans there is also another old saying: "Each moment of grief carves me deeper so I can contain more joy."

— Allen Rossman MD —

Dr. Allen Rossman is a practicing ophthalmologist whom I met shortly after he opened a practice in our community. That was 1978. For all these intervening years I have remembered the misfortune that befell him soon after his arrival. That memory has been highlighted by the fact that when he got sick the situation was so serious everyone thought he was going to die in a matter of weeks or months. The fact that he is still with us thirty years later is testament to the fact that a death sentence from cancer is not always carried out. And that fact is why I think you will get something out of this story too. I told this to Allen when I told him about this book and asked if we could get together and discuss his experience. Again, because of our first-hand acquaintance, I use his first name.

Allen had gone to Johns Hopkins for medical school. He took his specialty training at Yale then returned to the west coast where he had grown up. The culmination of his residency training he remembers as being a four-month stint working in a hospital clinic in Haiti.

So when Allen started having night sweats soon after starting his solo private practice, his first thought was, "Maybe I contracted tuberculosis in Haiti."

He went to one of the local internists who started a workup. The first thing was a battery of blood tests. Allen remembers the internist calling him the next day. It was right in the middle of office hours. He still remembers the words the other doctor spoke on the phone, "I'm coming over to see you." That alone was an alert about something serious being wrong. Allen recalls instantly having a feeling of dread. Less than an hour later Allen got the news face-to-face from the internist, "I think you have leukemia."

After that things moved very fast. Allen remembers his initial wave of despair. He smiles now recalling having a good cry with several other young, single physicians on the medical staff who had become his friends. He remembers some rumination about whether the stress of studying for his board certification might have left him vulnerable to such an illness. But there wasn't much time to reflect on anything. The word spread through the hospital staff that Allen had an extremely aggressive type of cancer, lymphoblastic leukemia. It was something usually found in children not adults. The prognosis was grim. Harrison's *Textbook of Medicine*, a standard text, had a statistic Allen looked up for himself. The textbook said he would be dead in six months. He told his parents the bad news and soon thereafter traveled to the University of Washington. He went to see the recommended medical oncologist, Dr. Fred Applebaum, at the Fred Hutchinson Cancer Center. He still counts himself lucky to have been put in the hands of someone both on the forefront of therapy and also a man whose personal interest and support became a mainstay over the years.

The initial therapy was extremely high doses of a steroid, Prednisone, followed by chemotherapies beginning with Vincristine. Without going into all those details he remembers so well, Allen summarized the attitude as being he was young and able to withstand a lot. The plan was to hit his cancer using a shotgun approach and use maximum dosages. Over time this meant the use of ten separate anti-tumor drugs in addition to the steroids.

He also remembers vividly the support from his family, especially visits from his father. When Allen's hair started to fall out in large patches, it was his father who went ahead and shaved the son's head.

Allen remembers the bone marrow biopsies. He endured them only with the aid of large injections of Demerol intravenously. He came to judge the competence of oncology fellows solely by the skill they demonstrated doing these procedures. "I had no idea what was going to happen to me, or how this was going to turn out," Allen recalls, "but I had great faith in Dr. Applebaum. I held onto the idea that I had to take responsibility. I didn't ever think this leukemia was my fault, but I knew instinctively that I would have to take responsibility for my care."

The field of bone marrow transplantation was still new. Much of the early work was done in Seattle at the Fred Hutchinson Center. The subject of this procedure came up as one of Allen's options. His feeling about this was not helped by attending a Grand Rounds where the presentation was the early clinical results of bone marrow transplants. The statistic he got at the time was one third of patients over 35 years old died outright from complications of the procedure. Failure from recurrences made success even more remote. Still, all the members of his family were tested. There was no acceptable tissue match found so no family member could donate bone marrow. Without a bone marrow match from the family and without the bone marrow banks available today, the only treatment was chemotherapy and radiation following the protocol prepared by Dr. Applebaum.

Allen gathered his facts from the point of view of being an ordinary patient. He was not feeling like a physician then. Not asking for any special consideration as a physician had its shortcomings in the hospital. Allen remembers lying freezing cold on a gurney in the x-ray department for long periods, waiting his turn for diagnostic procedures. It may not have amounted to special treatment, but Allen remembers his indwelling catheter used for chemotherapy, a Hickman catheter, was placed for him by its developer at the University, Dr. Hickman.

The protocol was to be with multiple anti-neoplastic agents given in combination instead of in sequence. After inducing remission, two courses of chemotherapy for near total destruction of the white cells were planned. This involved four different drugs for each course. The intent was to kill the more susceptible rapidly-dividing tumor cells, hopefully leaving some healthy bone marrow stock to repopulate the body. For a three-week period, with no functioning immune system, Allen was isolated in a laminar flow room, waiting for tests to confirm some normal cells were once again circulating in his blood.

Miserable with nausea, throat raw from a yeast infection (thrush), Allen was only able to eat mashed potatoes and soft boiled eggs. He remembers craving a tomato, but that was one of the things not allowed. He finally had to have hyper-alimentation for nutrition and also platelet transfusions to prevent bleeding.

Each of these immunosuppressive treatments was followed a week later by an unexplained fever. A workup included chest x-rays which revealed a spot on his upper right lung. After bronchoscopy and an unsuccessful attempt at biopsy, the consulting chest surgeon wanted to remove the upper lobe of Allen's right lung. This became a psychological low point. The chest surgeon's schedule was already full, after which he had plans to go out of town for Labor Day. He suggested to Allen that they wait until he returned. By the time the surgeon came back ready to operate, the shaking chills had mysteriously subsided. Repeat x-rays showed the suspicious spot on the lung had disappeared so surgery was avoided.

The Hickman catheter was suspected as a cause of the fevers and it was removed. Thereafter all infusions had to be made intravenously in the arms and other sites. This destroyed all the superficial veins, a problem which persists for Allen to this day. Because it was felt that the intravenous treatment might not cross the blood-brain barrier, Allen was given 5000 rads of radiation to his brain. He also had three courses of chemotherapy administered into the spinal fluid.

After the inpatient treatment an outpatient regimen of intravenous daunomycin, methotrexate, 6-mercaptopurine, and prednisone was devised. This continued once every twelve weeks for a total of twelve quarters, or three years. By mid-January of the next year, 1980, it was nearly seven months after diagnosis and Allen felt well enough to resume his clinical practice. He had quite a first year in practice!

Though he was still frightened after his experience and the prognosis, Allen felt bolstered by lots of outside support. He had come to know a half dozen oncologists and pathologists who played a role in his care. He became friends with all of them. He also had several girl friends before his treatment. He was pleased that one way or another, they all stuck with him during those difficult months. One of them, a young nurse, used to ride her bicycle some 20 miles along the Burke-Gilman trail in Seattle to visit while he was in University Hospital. Her effort to stay in contact impressed him very much at the time.

A year after diagnosis and back in his practice, a physician friend offered to introduce Allen to a nurse he knew who worked at a nearby community hospital. This was supposed to be a blind date, but when Allen asked the nurse, Debbie, out she said no. She finally agreed to go out, but only to lunch, not to dinner. Allen interpreted this as her wanting to be polite but not waste too much time on someone with cancer. He and everyone else knew he had a poor long-term prognosis. He thought she probably expected him to be dead soon.

Allen was immediately attracted to Debbie. She was both physically attractive and shared his sense of humor. They started dating regularly. Debbie had other talents. Because his date/nurse was skilled at starting an IV with a butterfly needle, she could administer his chemotherapy during the date if necessary!

While she gave the chemo, Debbie teased him. She began to speak of considering marriage. "You'll die soon. I'll inherit a rich doctor's fortune," she joked.

Not long after Allen and Debbie married. A month before their marriage in August, 1982, while still receiving the multi-drug treatment, Allen developed shingles (herpes zoster) on his scalp and neck. This was extremely painful and made him miserable. This was another low point. One doctor advised Allen nothing could be done and that the herpes could kill him. Another more knowledgeable physician told him of the new antiviral drug, acyclovir, and referred him back to the University Hospital. He received infusions of this new drug and recovered. He remembers feeling so thankful for medical progress.

Before the initial treatments had begun, Allen banked sperm knowing he would be sterile afterwards. Good fortune, however, allowed them to conceive two children in the normal fashion. When each of the two was born, Allen remembers, Debbie looked the infant over carefully then told her husband mischievously, "The baby looks just like your brother."

Allen had done some study of psychology before he got sick. He made his own assessment of himself. He tried to figure out what aspects of his life were not working. "What *runs me?*" he wanted to know. He made lists of issues he felt this way about. If he got angry he would remind himself that the source of that anger was within him, not in the situation itself. So, he would reason, "I have an option how to respond; I have a choice." Rather than blame others for anything he did not like, Allen made a change. He resolved to take responsibility for anything he himself could do. He learned to accept criticism. He refused to let it make him defensive. Allen feels this change is still a characteristic he has brought out of his ordeal. It is of benefit in his home life, his practice, and even in working with his staff.

Allen sees himself primarily as someone who has just stayed the course. He kept his practice of ophthalmology open and still enjoys it. "This is who I am," he told me. On many occasions Allen has been called upon by his oncologist friends to speak to cancer patients beginning chemotherapy. "Just stay the course," he advises these people, "It's not pleasant, but you can be optimistic that treatment will do you some good. Your chance to survive treatment is almost certain. So, I say, 'Go for it!'"

About ten years ago Allen was diagnosed as having hepatitis C. This almost certainly came from the pooled platelets he received during the initial cancer treatment. He tried interferon. His viral titer went down but he suffered a terrible autoimmune response with arthritis. He had to stop treatment. Because of the hepatitis C he knows he is at increased risk for developing liver cancer sometime in the future.

An additional health issue is a hereditary condition, medullary sponge kidney. At least he has known about this one since the time of medical school. It has caused episodes of pain and the most serious of those was in mid-1982 while still taking treatment. In addition to everything else that was going on, he simultaneously passed a stone from each kidney. This was the most painful experience of Allen's life and was complicated even further by development of a serious kidney infection. Both of the stones had to be surgically removed.

So still there are reminders of the past. But the diagnosis of lymphoblastic leukemia was made 28 years ago. The prognosis then was six months. His marriage, his family, his career in ophthalmology have all come after that. His conclusion is, "Take things day by day. Go ahead and make plans for the future. Neither you nor I are going to die next week. So, you need a plan."

— JAMES G. MHYRE MD —

James G. Mhyre, MD, became a partner in my surgical clinic in 1980. We had daily contact in clinical practice for many years. We became friends and have remained in frequent contact since I retired from practice. Through our ongoing relationship I came to know of a personal ordeal that Dr. Mhyre lived through several years ago. I saw some of it, but that was only the outside. Jim did not have cancer, but his story is another good one. It's about how a physician, in this case a general surgeon, deals with life-threatening illness. Dr. Mhyre is back in practice now. His outcome will give you additional insight as to how surgeons think. You will learn something from this additional facet of illness. Jim always has been a keen observer. This was such a good story when he recounted it to me that I asked him to write it himself. This is what he gave me.

I would like to present a surgical case, my own. In addition to being a general surgeon, I also have been a surgical patient. The following tale will illustrate a few points about human nature. It will also give a rationale for something I believe in, the use of the electronic personal health record or PHR.

Up until a few years ago my personal health was normal, routine, and even dull. I do have a few skeletons in my family history closet such as my father dying at my current age from a myocardial infarction. I take a hand full of vitamins, 81 mg of aspirin, and a statin to keep my cholesterol around 180. My recent colonoscopy and PSA were normal. I always took it for granted that my health had been normal, was normal today, and will be normal tomorrow. If I had had a PHR, it would have been basic, sparse, and relatively static over time.

That all changed one evening in 2003. I was taking ER call from home. I was doing some home repairs with plastic putty containing a strong smelling solvent. The fumes gave me a headache and made me nauseated. I lay down for 10 minutes and my symptoms improved. I got up and resumed working with the strong solvent. The symptoms recurred, this time even worse. I do a lot of wood working but had not experienced anything like that before. I also felt malaise, nausea with diaphoresis, and vertigo. I had an odd ache behind my right eye which I had trouble ignoring. I felt like crap and decided just to lie down and go to sleep. Then my pager went off.

Calls from the ER are usually unwelcome and this was a typical one of those: it sounded like another person with appendicitis. I muttered a response to the inquiry about how soon I could get in there. I rallied enough to get to my car. Once seated I did not feel too badly driving the 10 miles up the freeway provided I did not move my head. At the hospital I got through the ER patient's evaluation and confirmed the diagnosis. About that time it dawned on me maybe I couldn't make it through doing an appendectomy. Maybe I should admit the patient and start antibiotics. I could get some sleep. I would feel better in the morning.

While I sat at the work desk thinking about these options the ER doctor saw me. He told me later I was pale and sweaty and holding my head. He asked me a few questions then suggested I go lie down on a gurney. He wanted to order a CT scan on me. If you are a medical diagnostician reading this you will have a pretty good idea what was happening to me. At that moment my power of denial did not allow me even to have a differential diagnosis to consider. I still assumed I was sick from the solvent fumes.

The CT was done promptly. It demonstrated a posterior fossa hemorrhage (bleeding into the cerebellum at the back of my brain). This proved to be from arterio-venous malformation (AVM) and a small aneurysm. Bleeding into the base of the brain is usually catastrophic. For some reason this time it was not fatal. The bleeding had stopped spontaneously. I was hospitalized and my symptoms improved over the next 24 hours. Who knows what would have happened if the ER had not called me in that night? What if, instead, I had stayed home and just gone to sleep?

Now my task was to select the right person to advise me on what to do. I had the advantage of insider knowledge and assistance from my partners in selecting the regional expert in AVMs at our nearby academic medical center.

An AVM is a structural problem. We needed an accurate map of the vascular anatomy. The CT angiogram was not detailed enough. This meant a six-vessel cerebral angiogram. I foolishly wanted to experience what this more traditional test felt like. I cavalierly declined any sedation. That was a very bad idea. Once the injection catheter was in place the radiologist retreated to his radiation-proof control room. He engaged the automatic power injector to commence firing. Each salvo of dye slamming into my brain generated a 10 second pseudo-psychedelic burst. Suddenly I experienced a terrible stabbing pain in my neck. I did not think of vasospasm. My reaction was that the catheter had gone into the wall of the vessel and was creating a carotid artery dissection! This is a complication of angiograms where the inner lining of the artery strips away from the outer wall and can block off blood flow entirely. Was I about to get a stroke from just having a test? I wiggled my hands and feet to see if I could tell which part was being paralyzed first. I made a feeble attempt to call out for help. All that brought was a response over the loudspeakers. A booming voice commanded, "HOLD STILL!" Clearly the radiology crew was on a mission. The mission was to get sharp pictures, not to have a conversation with me.

With these additional results in hand my consulting neurosurgeon evaluated all options. I remember thinking how many times I had gone through this deliberative process, only then I was the decision-maker and someone else, not me, was the patient. The neurosurgeon considered the likelihood of success, the risks (including loss of my life), complications such as stroke, cost, what the literature recommended, along with available technology and expertise. He delivered his recommendations to me, the patient. It was up to me to sign off on the strategy, in spite of my limited understanding and clouded thinking.

What it came down to was, for an AVM in a 56 year old, there are three choices: observe only, attack with cold steel, or go nuclear! Observation is too risky; re-bleed is likely and could be fatal. Surgery eliminates the problem directly and is definitive if the technical part is successful. It carries, however, a higher upfront risk of both morbidity and mortality. Radio surgery is the third and newer option. Here either a linear accelerator or Cobalt-60 acts as the energy source and irradiates the AVM in a single session. The other choice here is the Gamma Knife with a mortality of 1% and morbidity of 3%. It is painless and there is little recovery time. With the Gamma Knife it takes one to three years to shrivel up and obliterate the AVM. That leaves some exposure to re-bleeding at any moment during that time span. Also, it is only 80 to 90% effective. My neurosurgeon and I both favored surgery. We were both biased toward physical methods and definitive outcomes. I did not like the long latency time and uncertain success with the Gamma Knife.

I was transferred for another hospitalization, this time under the care of the local interventional neuroradiology guru at the medical center. This was for embolization of the posterior inferior cerebellar artery which is where the trouble lay. This second angiogram went much smoother as I was under general anesthesia, a wise choice for everyone involved. After having as much blood flow blocked as possible, I was ready for surgery.

This was the first time I can recall riding a gurney into the operating room where I was not in command and in control. At least my surgical team made me feel comfortable and I had confidence in them. My next six hours were spent lying face down. My skull was screwed into a bracket and that was bolted to the frame of the table. My cerebellum was exposed by first detaching the large muscles on the back of my neck. After that a two-inch disc of bone from the base of my skull behind those muscles was removed. Several cubic centimeters of my cerebellum brain tissue were scooped out, along with the cluster of abnormal blood vessels. Tiny metal clips were used to occlude all surrounding vessels. Two days later I woke up. I was in a private room in the neurosurgery ward. I realized how lucky I was to have been out of it for a couple of days while I was intubated and sedated. That was good but I was not prepared for what came next.

The vertigo, the dizziness associated with working on that part of my brain, was severe. Everything in the room was spinning even with my lying flat in bed. Each of my eyes had a mind of its own and spun independent of the other. My right eye began doing a rock 'n roll while the left one tried break dancing. Meanwhile the entire hospital room kept tipping over and over, end over end. I was doing what felt like an aerial dogfight; I was darting and dodging, climbing and diving, twisting and turning for nearly a week. I ran through the entire pharmacopoeia of drugs but the nausea remained disabling. Temporary relief came only after throwing up and I did that day and night.

Slowly central command, that is, the rest of my brain, reestablished some control. My eyes quit going their separate ways and the double vision cleared. I still had bursts of nystagmus (where the eyes track laterally, back and forth, back and forth) and vertigo, but all this gradually became less intense. The hospital food began to stay down. By the eighth postoperative day I felt good enough to declare victory. I gave my thanks to the staff for their commitment and hard work. I was very sincere about that. Then I headed home.

The warmest memory of that hospitalization was a male nurse. He took extra time to communicate with me on a personal level. He gave repeated assurances that the nystagmus, vertigo, and nausea would eventually stop. Intellectually I already knew what he was saying. Now in my role as the patient, his words were very reassuring. He was an exceptional caregiver and I appreciated all that he did. I was relieved to be able to walk out of there. I was still unsteady and needed a walker to keep from falling over but I was determined to leave under my own power. As I awkwardly rolled my walker ahead of me I did feel a few drops roll down the back of my neck. They trickled down between my shoulder blades. Sweat, I thought.

Coming home took some adjustment. First I had to allow myself to be cared for and pampered by my wife. This wasn't easy. Personal dependency does not come naturally to me. Karen is a trained nurse. She did a wonderful job helping me through this and putting up with my crankiness. Second I had to learn how to rest. That does not come naturally either. Normally I wake up around 5:30 and cannot sleep past 6:00 even if I want to. After being away from the pressures of practice and early morning hospital meetings for a few weeks, I actually started sleeping in! Sometimes I did not wake up until eight o'clock. I could never sleep in before that time, or since, for that matter.

I still had some cerebellar dysfunction to get through. I was noticeably ataxic (where my limbs and digits would not agree to do what I told them). That was worse on the left side than the right. Fortunately I am right-handed. I put away my walker after a week at home. I was still having bouts of vertigo but thankfully they were no longer accompanied by nausea. I started thinking about when I could get back to work. Was my cognitive function diminished? Would this trouble in using my left side remain? My patients' safety had to be my first concern. I knew I would lose patients' confidence if my attempt at eye contact was disrupted by my eyeballs flicking back and forth from one wall of an exam room to the other. Should I advise my staff to reopen my schedule? When could I start seeing office patients? As it turned out I need not have worried about resuming practice just then.

In neurosurgery circles, a drop of "sweat" trickling down the neck of a post op craniotomy patient means fluid around the brain is leaking out. This is a big deal, even an emergency! I had this brain fluid, or cerebrospinal fluid (CSF), leak and didn't know it. It provided an avenue for infection and eventually, meningitis. About two weeks after arriving home I began feeling poorly. I had a fever again. A few days later I was so incapacitated that my wife had to call 911 to get me out of the house. Back in the hospital a drain catheter was put back in my spine to vent the dangerous buildup in fluid pressure. I remained in the hospital for 10 days getting high-dose antibiotics for meningitis. Over the next month while I continued on IV antibiotics at home my symptoms gradually went away.

I resumed my original recovery trajectory. My cerebellar symptoms, the dizziness, subsided to where they were bothersome but not disruptive. I went back to work seeing patients and doing surgery. Frequently I had an infusion pump hanging around my neck under my sterile gown infusing antibiotics.

Then the low grade fevers returned again. My other symptoms returned and slowly I began to deteriorate. I had yet another hospitalization. I continued to have white cells in my CSF as evidence of another infection around my brain. The cycles of sweats and chills intensified. Nothing was working. I tried to prepare myself for progressive central nervous system infection and a bad outcome.

After three months of deteriorating strength and continuing fevers I was back in the operating room. It was my second major procedure. I was feeling both lousy and pessimistic. This time the disk of bone covering the original surgery site and my brain was found to be the cause of infection and removed. The wound was irrigated and the bone defect bridged with a titanium mesh screwed into the surrounding skull. My neck muscles were reattached to the mesh. This was a desperate situation and pretty much a last ditch thing to do, putting hardware like that in an infected space. But it worked!

After another 6 weeks of antibiotics, I was finally clear of infection. The total campaign lasted five months. It included four CT scans, two angiograms, two major surgeries, six hospitalizations at three different hospitals, four spinal taps, and four months of self-administered antibiotics through a central catheter. My professional staff included two neurosurgeons, two ER physicians, six different radiologists, four anesthesiologists (one of my buddies did a spinal tap for me), two infectious disease specialists, one hospitalist, and body parts were examined by two pathologists. There was an additional legion of residents, fellows, rounding partners, pharmacists, and other professionals of various stripes also involved. My insurance company paid nearly all of the cost of $130,000! My regular physician did not find out about any of this until it was all over. He was out of the loop because no one thought to tell him.

I had to make a decision regarding disability. I had lost about 10 cubic centimeters of my cerebellum and there were consequences to that. I had lost considerable physical conditioning and strength. I had to watch carefully when I walked to keep from staggering noticeably like I was drunk. I was prone to bursts of vertigo, especially when I looked up. I had lost some coordination in my left hand, a potentially significant disability for a surgeon. I was not sure about cogitative function but felt I was thinking clearly. Should I apply for disability and receive monthly payments from my insurance carrier for the next 8 years? I had had two separate surgical recovery periods, neither lasting the requisite three months to trigger my disability insurance. My ongoing monthly overhead at the office and lost productivity had to be covered. Should I attempt to resurrect my surgical career? Would I recover sufficiently to operate safely? I could make a legitimate case either way.

These were the things going through my mind at the time. In the end I felt I was not ready to identify myself as disabled. I wanted to continue to be a practicing surgeon. I requested a statement from my neurosurgeon assuring my hospital's credentials committee it was safe for me to resume practice. I went to work and in another month was back in the OR on the handle end of a knife.

Where am I now, three years later? I still think about this experience all the time. I have a perceptible clumsiness in my left hand. I feel the same way when I walk across anything other than a flat, completely open floor. I get dizzy easily. I still have vertigo briefly when I look up. My neck muscles tug on the mesh at the base of my skull. I can still feel the sensation. When that happens it pulls on the linings around my brain and on the cerebellum scar underneath; that stimulates an attack of vertigo. I can perform surgery without compromise as long as I am careful doing things like looking up to adjust the OR light. I have never regained my pre-surgical physical conditioning. Is it because I'm getting old? Did the neurosurgery impact me more than I realize? Or am I just not trying hard enough?

I consider myself healthy—well, pretty healthy. And, maybe I work too hard and don't sleep enough. Maybe I still eat too much, and stress out too often, and don't get enough exercise, and drink too much coffee. I actually have gotten busier approaching retirement. I have taken on a number of administrative positions as well as my surgery practice. To maintain balance I've limited myself to working just half time. (Half time to a surgeon is 84 hours a week.) One of these days things will slow down. Then I will have more time for my family and my own health. For now, there is just too much to do.

I live with some occupational hazards that I have dodged so far. My cumulative radiation exposure may catch up with me some day. I come in daily contact with all types of nasty infections and secretions and blood. Universal precautions reduce the risk but there are still needle sticks and

cuts. I have two colleagues who had to give up surgery after they contracted hepatitis C.

I ask myself, is stress and its accompanying adrenalin rush the spice of
life? Or is it the agent of death? For a general surgeon stress comes with
the territory. Every now and then I have a big adrenalin surge when blood
splashes in my face or when I sense sweat running down my back. How do
we know when awareness becomes fear? Surgeons get used to operating
on people or they change careers. I know I am more comfortable entering someone's personal space in the operating room then I am entering
their personal space at a social gathering. More stressful is the state of
uncertainty when a patient is deteriorating out of control and they have
entrusted me to solve their problem. What is causing the problem in their
abdomen or chest cavity? Does their life depend on my assessment, my decisions in the next few minutes? Will that person die without an operation?
Are they strong enough to survive surgery? Sometimes an unknown evil
force seems to be at work. Am I being too complacent? Uncertainty wears
on me as much as making an overt mistake.

Ultimate stress is when a major complication occurs or my patient dies.
This is especially true if what happens is unexpected. I feel in my own moments of self-criticism that I could have, and should have, performed better.
Was I distracted? Did I not try hard enough? Was I choosing expediency
over safety? Recovering from this emotion and guilt can take weeks. It can
take years if lawyers get involved. There are several studies in the literature
reporting higher rates of burnout or early retirement, plus suicide, divorce,
alcoholism, and drug abuse among surgeons compared to other professionals. I have dodged all of those bullets so far too. My candle is burning brightly but definitely on both ends. I know it. I have to assume that part of the cost
of being a surgeon is two or three years of my own life being squandered
through stress. I have not seen any reports of shortened life expectancy for
surgeons, but it would follow that if high stress is bad, I cannot expect to live
as long as if I had chosen some other profession. Maybe I should have gone
into health care planning and gotten a masters in public health. Maybe I
could have been an insurance company CEO with an MBA. Is it possible to
write off the monetary value of a couple of years of my life to stress on my
income taxes? I do it for my other business expenses!

I have made a career working with the ill and the dying. I was very
fortunate to have survived a serious medical threat to my own life. I am
turning 60. What's coming next and when will it come? From which direc-

tion will the next attack be launched? Will the first assault be something I fail to recognize? Will it be an annoying harassment or the beginning of a prolonged siege? Or will the attack on my well-being be overwhelmingly forceful and decisive? Maybe covert operatives are attacking this very minute, working silently to soften my defenses.

I wait … and watch … and wonder!

Will it be ASCVD, MI, COPD, CVA, MS, Tb, ALS, SLE, HIV, CLL, AML? These are just some of the arcane medical acronyms we use as labels. Maybe what attacks me will be perforated diverticulitis, necrotizing fasciitis, or biliary pancreatitis. I bet I will get CANCER some day! Will it be prostate, pancreas, lung, or colon? Will I need a radical prostatectomy, a pancreaticoduodenectomy, a total pneumonectomy, a coloproctectomy, a trisegmental hepatectomy or some other technically challenging operative procedure done on me?

Maybe I'll get a viral cardiomyopathy. In that case I will need a good chronic disease program for my congestive heart failure. Will the final beats of my heart be my own heart, or will it be someone else's heart that has been transplanted in my chest? Will I have a colostomy, an ileostomy, or a urostomy to change my daily life routine? I do not want to die of bowel obstruction! Will I be incontinent? That would be preferable, of course, to no urine at all. I don't want to have dialysis three times a week. Will I suffer? Will I be in pain? Will my legs require new hip or knee joints to continue functioning? Will I even continue to have legs? I could not cope with paralysis like quadriplegia but that's possible considering what has happened to me before. Will I get depressed, suicidal, paranoid, or psychotic? Will I be able to hear my favorite music, to see, to read, to think? Will I still recognize my family? I'm afraid that thirty years in medicine has altered my perspective and jaded my soul. Maybe everything will continue to work just fine well into old age…before it all shuts down at once! To me, that is health care's most perfect outcome!

What do I need to strengthen my defenses? First, I need the support of my family. We are all interconnected and my illnesses are theirs. I need knowledgeable and skilled professionals to help me. My own experience will not be sufficient. My medical judgment is inherently flawed when applied to myself or my family's health decisions. I will need access to money, mine or society's, to fund my health care. To help me communicate with my physicians, and organize my health information I have come to believe

I need my own personal health record. I see different doctors at various times but I live with my health problems all of the time!

It is up to me to muster whatever resources I can to put up a defense. Ultimately, I am the one responsible for my own health and well being. In the coming years we will all need our own personal health record (PHR). That one thing will allow us to exchange information, and our thoughts, with our physicians in standardized ways. My personal health record is my record of my own self. It is not something belonging even to my personal physician. It certainly does not belong to the electronic record of some other entity like an insurance company or hospital or Microsoft. The medication list in my PHR is my official medication list. My private physician and any specialists I see may keep a dated copy of my medication list in his electronic record because I permit it, not the other way around.

We are all on our own journeys through life. To some extent we have a shared destiny. Personal health records will at least help make the medical aspects of these journeys more efficient and healthy. This is what I'm working to make practical now.

I will not go gentle into that good night … but I know I will go. I will have a plan to maximize the calculus of my life, the integral of function over time. I will also have a plan to minimize my suffering. My physicians may be ethically conflicted but my family and I are clear and less constrained in applying wisdom and common sense. I doubt that I have the resolve to do some heroic thing but when the time comes, I will make my end of life directives clearly known through the use of my personal health record.

CHAPTER 10

THE TASK OF RENEWING OURSELVES

I asked God, "How long do I have to live?"
God answered, "Long enough to make a difference."
— *Anonymous*

You cannot do a kindness too soon, for you never know
how soon it will be too late.
— *Ralph Waldo Emerson*

Identifying a cause for cancer has been difficult. Theories about causation are countless. Hypotheses about targeting a cure are everywhere and, certainly, finding a general solution has been elusive. At the same time anything that brings about healing or relieves suffering is imminently practical. There is no cure for cancer here and the healing process is mostly internal work hidden from view. Hopefully these stories from Renewal help reveal your unique path to discovery and healing without promising cure.

Since about 2001 an attractive new idea called the cancer stem cell hypothesis has been gaining credibility. In essence it says that all tissues have stem cells, or progenitor cells that act the same way. When these cells are damaged and begin to propagate tumors, they divide into two, but only one becomes a cancer cell. The other daughter cell remains a stem cell like its parent. This daughter continues on making two new cells, another stem cell like itself and one cancer cell. So over time the tumor has two separate populations. When medical treatment is applied to kill the cancer cells, and we see a tumor diminished in size by radiation or chemotherapy, the stem cell population may not be as susceptible. The stem cells survive to continue propagating. If these observations are correctly interpreted, the opportunity to devise treatments for the stem cell line presents itself.

Another new development in cancer research is an outgrowth of sequencing the human genome. Specific gene abnormalities have been found to be associated with certain tumors. The cost of analyzing a person's genetic makeup has been falling rapidly, but these analyses still are complicated. This complexity poses a problem in terms of how to apply this knowledge to whole populations. In other words, how can the science in this be used in detection and preventive medicine?

The Institute for Systems Biology in Seattle may have an answer. Each of the 60 organs in our bodies produces a molecule specific to that organ. These molecules circulate in the blood as biomarkers of their site of origin. These can be detected in extremely small amounts; all 60 can be identified in less than a drop of blood. So if a blood sample is taken and assayed when someone is young, results can be used to predict the probability of developing an organ-specific abnormality later in life, like cancer of the ovary. Each person serves as their own control. An assay in later life can be compared to earlier results. If tests indicate the biomarker from a certain organ is changing, investigation is carried out to determine if a cancer in a pre-clinical stage is developing.

Thoughts of such scientific developments can become exhilarating. That may be, but you may not feel you have the luxury of waiting for practical applications of research to reveal themselves. The assumption of this final chapter is that the reader will be best served with a discussion of how to get mentally prepared to meet your challenges, not a survey of the field of cancer research.

Many magazines and books sell themselves by promoting lists for self-improvement. This may be about losing weight, how to sleep all night, have great sex, or anything else we think we want. It is my belief that such lists, even when factually correct, are rarely acted upon by the reader. Thus they have little impact. On the other hand stories we can relate to do have impact upon the human brain, more so than persuasive arguments or even what is reported as scientific fact. That's just the way humans are wired. Some recent evidence suggests the brain actually is able to reconfigure genes, so there is a lot more to learn about what our thinking influences. What you have been presented in preceding chapters is a number of true stories about people with cancer and about the group support we all received in Renewal meetings.

At the end, in the Appendices, are summaries of basic first steps suggested for you to take with diet and strengthening your body. There is also a list of books recommended by Renewal. These books will be helpful if you are looking for something more to read. The first appendix and the bulk of this present chapter deal with the all-important issue of your mental state, your attitude, and your willingness to help your self. Laurence Gonzales says in his book *Deep Survival* if we only follow medical advice or our intellect, we cut ourselves off from our bodies and our emotions. He says the body controls the brain just as much as the brain controls the body.

Important now is what your assessment of self reveals and your coming to terms with who you are. Your situation needs to mesh with your developing conviction, clarity of purpose, and determination for self-improvement. Our group came to call the many ramifications of this process Renewal. What you call it is up to you. As someone once told us, the antidote for tiredness is not rest; the antidote for tiredness is **wholeheartedness.**

Courage, heroism, persistence, are all terms most Renewal members deflect from themselves with a self-conscious smile. Let's just acknowledge that they are a group of people, from teenagers to some in their nineties, all wearing a label affixed by the medical establishment. They are called cancer patients or cancer victims. Renewal members analyze their present situation and decide there is something more. They peel off those old labels or apply new ones more of their own choosing. Some Renewal members want more *time* with family, to go back and fill old holes in their relationships. Some want to *accomplish something* or complete some undertaking. Some want to find *happiness* or *contentment,* elusive things that have escaped them. Some just want to *continue on in life* for a while longer, having focus now on a new goal or having a clearer purpose.

The stories about Renewal members earlier in the book were chosen as facets of truth about illness and healing. None are distorted or contrived. As a reader your time to act is now, while these stories are fresh in your mind. Today is a gift; that's why we call it The Present. A new application of The Present can start when you put this book down.

There never was a formula for Renewal. The process relies upon stories, along with mutual support and sharing in general. Based upon what we have done and what follows in the remainder of this book, it is my hope that you will decide upon a renewal of your own. By now the resourcefulness and resilience of our members are self-evident. Our members can serve as your model. We will show you how these lessons can be adopted directly by you or someone you know in need of assistance.

Let's begin this way: if you want to start a physical fitness program or lose weight, you will be wise to hire an experienced trainer. If you ask your trainer what to expect, you likely will hear a prediction that goes something like this: It's your mental attitude that will change first, not something observable. You will get tired as you work, then feel new abilities begin to appear. After that you will feel your body changing and develop a new confidence. Next comes demonstrable new strength and flexibility. An observable shift in bodily proportions follows and if it is weight loss you want, that will come last. In other words, after you decide to become something different, it's mental attitude that changes first. Reaching a goal comes later.

Frank G. Burgess said, "Our bodies are apt to be our autobiographies," It's time to start writing your own script.

Being in a support group like Renewal can take you a long way. Even this book telling about Renewal will provide enough to get started. Remember, wherever your journey is beginning, one path will never take you all the way to the end. More exploration and concomitant change will be necessary. Intellectual pursuits alone will not lead to where you want to be. The majority of what you want comes only from experience. What you decide to do about your treatment, conventional or unconventional, will take care of the physical part. What we add in these pages is to take care of the spiritual part.

Not only will the beginning path not take you all the way, the path is never straight. Like the design on the cover of this book, your life path takes turns. Something new lies over the hill, hidden from view. You cannot see it. Your task now is to choose to walk on the path immediately in front of you.

Remember too, trying to be a "good" patient carries with it an element of ego. If I am a good patient I'll have a better chance of being accepted in this strange land of medical care. The notion is if I am good I will be rewarded. Forget about rewards. Ego binds you to justifying what has worked for you in the past, to having been right. Use new information and experiences to change your mental model and the map of where you go. Forget about who you were and about being right. Forget ego. Creativity limited by ego will limit options and prevent your growth.

Forgiveness has been put forth repeatedly as the way to unburden your self for this new journey. It is metaphorically the key to the lock. The lock in turn represents what is keeping a door inside you from opening. That door has a duality. What lies beyond both frightens and excites us. We are blocked in our progress and don't know what lies on the other side. Going through any psychological passageway like this causes mixed emotions. It's a very difficult thing to do. The path to anything new exposes our vulnerability. One day you will know what you have to do. Take that new path.

Forgiveness is to start over again with truthfulness. It wipes away the diaphanous web entangling you with evasions and half-truths. Being truthful allows you to be authentic. Being authentic gives you strength. Strength makes you courageous. Courage provides resolve to work through your problems. With work you learn persistence. As you stay with your inner work, seeing progress will lead to love of what you are doing. As love expands it becomes unselfish. Unselfish love will engage you in service and service is strongly associated with survival. At this stage of refinement your path will roll out before you. You move closer to being what you want to be and merge with your destiny. You establish the value of your new life and regain control.

We are saying test the potential of who you can be. I've added, "Be realistic," but at the same time have tried to avoid using the admonition, "be reasonable." Being reasonable is often the old, cautious you. It connotes the limits others expect and their judgments. Look for creative ways to express your true self. As you nurture and care for your self, look for any roadblocks developing along the path to continued progress. This will be the place to cycle through forgiveness again.

What helps us move ahead is our surrender. This surrender has nothing to do with accepting defeat. It is surrender to our situation and vulnerability of being on a different and novel path. Following a new way is more likely to take us where we want to be. This is another instance where a group approach like Renewal can help. Empathetic voices join our new conversation with ourselves. We put down the weight of our aloneness and join others in common cause.

It is true that we ultimately are alone in life, but it is a mistake to undertake the struggle with illness alone. Warning: Be prepared to receive some negative responses when you share the new self you are creating. What you are experiencing inside cannot be seen by everyone else. It is axiomatic that personal growth is not a spectator sport. See words of discouragement or being rebuffed as a gift. Negative feedback from family and acquaintances help clarify relationships. Being excluded in one place may force you to seek new allies elsewhere. If it becomes necessary to make choices, do not give in to the old way. Move forward on your own.

Coach John Wooden said, "Don't let what you can't do interfere with what you can do." And Herm Albright (1876-1944) gave a bit of mischievous advice when he said, "A positive attitude may not solve all your problems, but it will annoy enough people to make it worth the effort."

In childhood our path presented many options. Remember how you daydreamed about adult life and doing grown-up things? Can you conceive of your present situation having possibilities like that? Is it possible to daydream again? This is where guided meditation and the creativity of drawing can assist you. If you pose questions now you will discover the blessing hidden inside the trials of illness. New answers will come and lead you on. If you turn away from your questions they do not disappear. Any time you pause and look back, any unresolved issues will still be there, following you and waiting for attention.

A disease like cancer can be the unanswered questions in life. It presents uncertainty personified. Disease, like jumbled questions and wrong answers, interrupts what you are doing and stops what you are becoming. Ask the important questions. What is my purpose? What is my mission in life? How do I accomplish my goals? And get your priorities straight. Don't deal with trivialities when your life is on the line. Don't let procedural decisions unmake your life.

If you have trouble constructing your goals, try subtraction or reducing the options. One useful exercise you can do for your self starts with listing the ten most important things in your life. Go ahead. Put all ten on separate sheets of paper. What matters most in my life? When you have done that, consider each of your choices. Discard the one you consider least important. Crumple that sheet and throw it away. Think about the meaning of abandoning that choice. Next, consider the remaining nine and again discard the least important of those remaining. Continue this process until only one sheet of paper with one value remains. Each choice you make narrows the deliberation and makes remaining choices more intense.

People starting this exercise often have "Being alive" or similar sentiments among their ten choices. Usually that turns out not to be the last one remaining. In other words, participants will define something else as more important than life itself. What is that something for you? Whatever accomplishment or relationship survives this winnowing process moves to the top. It is your new primary reason for fighting to live.

We speak of healing rather than of cure. You need to ponder the difference. Getting well can mean healing as well as the cure you probably are thinking about. You need to achieve peace of mind to make significant progress. Peace of mind or contentment, acceptance or surrender in the volitional sense, are all ways to describe the goal and the route that takes you there.

Spirituality cannot be taught, it must be experienced. The unconscious mind is far more creative than the conscious mind. This is why intellectual pursuits, the study, the thinking about your illness, are only the superficial commitments to getting well. Our mind, our intellect, is always analyzing, always hypothesizing. It never stops, even when we sleep. To benefit from the mind we educate it, use it as a resource, and ask it questions, but realize its limitations: Our spirit, our soul, is the silent part of us that lies beyond the mind. The soul needs no education. It needs instead to have an opening prepared, like cutting away brush in a forest and clearing a space separate from the trees. Once we have created a suitable opening for the soul we have to wait. Our purpose eventually will emerge from the silence and gloom among those trees.

The spiritual realm is vast but it is not trackless. Look for signs left by the wisdom of others as you search. Correct paths will have many footprints. If what you discover makes sense to you, follow those footprints as a guide for your own journey. Study what has illuminated lives through the ages. One caution: if you feel satisfied with your past good works and present belief system, the prayers made up to this moment, you may be certain you have not done enough yet.

Life is a continuing conversation with self. It is not an exercise in command and control. We need to understand our mortality. Pat W. is remembered in Renewal for uttering her famous realization to us, "My cancer may kill me, but it has healed my life!" Having cancer gives you the right to ponder this strange utterance and what it means. Once we understand, we need never stand at this same threshold of indecision again.

Serious illness is the time our efforts produce the most benefit, but not necessarily the results we wait for. We need to have the will to call our spirit back. Part of us is being consumed, used up and exhausted by the chatter of everyday life. In the past, part of our energy flowed out into things like our profession or raising children. Now you need to marshal this energy to contend with disease and treatment. If you feel you never found a purpose in life, one is now being thrust before you. The contest will be difficult. It brings to mind a poem in Rainer Maria Rilke's *The Book for the Hours* (also called Das Studenbuch) quoted here in part:

> *I am pushing through solid rock*
> *in flint like layers, as the ore lies, alone;*
> *I am such a long way in I see no way through,*
> *and no space; everything is close to my face,*
> *and everything close to my face is stone...*
> *...You see, I want a lot*
> *Perhaps I want everything.*

This is the work, part physical but mostly mental. You may be unaccustomed to such sustained effort. This exploration seems at first to be something only involving the intellect. Here is a place where persistence is valuable, but I advise you to reassess frequently how much your physical strength will allow. Prudence may require you to go slowly, though that certainly wasn't the case with Margaret P., was it? She said she would do everything to get well, not just negotiate with her cancer. You may have to wait until treatment is over to start renewing your self. Or, like Bill W. with his radiation, and as others in Renewal viewed their chemo or surgery, treatment may be what you see as taking the old you and putting it to a torch. You may decide to rebuild, to renew your self and only ashes of the old you remain. There is a message left if you extinguish the former you in this way. Bend over and see what message is written in the dust of those ashes for you to understand.

There was nothing about Renewal that advocated ignoring pain and anxiety. Pain is an obstacle to your progress. It needs to be dealt with. Use medication when appropriate. Remember balance even if you forget being reasonable about your illness; this is not a place for bravado. In our group conversations we tried to explore things for what they meant, to process challenges, then combine our individual talents to endure and prevail. Realize that the greatest pain for you may be psychic not physical, like the woman with the son in prison mentioned in Chapter 1. Such psychic pain comes from many sources. These include the experience of realizing the distance, the separation, between who we are now from who we want to be.

We have not said much about the whole body of work that exists concerning the subject of change. Some people find it easier to label this process a transition, not change. It's an interesting subject but probably peripheral to what you need at this point. You probably say, "I don't want to change. I just want to get the old me back!" and that's a legitimate goal. It is certainly one of the choices on the path toward healing—just realize it may not be a practical option. What is an option is the choice to use your period of illness, awful and protracted as it may be, as a teachable moment. This is the suggestion of the last few pages. This very moment is the time to emerge as more than you were before. Effort, persistence, unpredictability and uncertainty about outcome are the hallmarks of choosing a new path.

Change can be an easy concept to accept if you fully explore it. It can be the currency you use to pay for the voyage to a new you. Change in the context of physical renewal is important but incomplete. Change needs to happen at the level where a problem is being experienced. To say it another way, change is not a broad and unfocused mantra for being different for unspecified reasons. This is not like a business enterprise going through retooling to prepare for a new production line. It is not analogous to hiring a new CEO to be a change agent for two or three years only to clean house then be replaced. What change you choose to make is integral to the work you do. Having said that, once you start changing, you may decide to change everything.

In the midst of illness you need peace of mind. If you are too disturbed by your illness, too frightened, you will not hear the alternatives, the opportunities, when they are presented to you. Stress causes us to make mistakes. You will see more options when you feel better. Continue the inner work while doing the outer work. Make your assessment of what your personal priorities are and map them out. Get started on a mental map, a plan.

Change is a bit like setting out in a sail boat. First you set an objective and plot a course to begin the voyage. You use the energy of the wind to drive in one direction, then tack to use the wind to go back the other way. Each time you make a new calculation and set a new course. You make these adjustments, changing direction and position all along the trip, but the destination remains constant.

Set goals, short, medium, and long. Short is right now, what to do today, this week. This very day is The Present life has provided, so use it. What are your midrange goals? As a practical matter, most people with cancer have more time left to live than they initially assume. What are your long-term goals? Remember the member stories in Chapters 2 and 3. These people in Renewal were not optimistic at the start. Now, ten, twenty, thirty years later they still are here, making adjustments to deal with old age.

One thing to do is start making a list. You can begin today, but the process of compiling a list needs to continue long enough for you to really scour your brain for all your issues. There are several ways to do this. One is to put a line down the middle of a blank page and start two columns. One side is the positive things in your life and on the other side of the line, the negative. List people, accomplishments, resources, and attributes you have in both columns. It's like tabulating assets and liabilities. A similar separate list can be used for short-, medium- and long-term goals. List the things you want with what is keeping you from obtaining them.

A third type of list is the fun things you like to do. Include some things to schedule for fun each day. Yet another educational list is compiling the lessons learned from your illness. What thoughts about the world around you have been altered since receiving your diagnosis?

Keeping a journal is a good idea. There are whole books on how to do it if you want step-by-step instruction. Keep things simple as you start out. Here are a few reasons to actually do this: One is, if you start writing, you can leave a chronology for your family about this unique journey you are taking. Consider how many people care about you and are in this with you—even if they never have told you so. Think how much they want to know about your thoughts and what you are learning but don't know how to ask. Your thinking may be muddled now or at some time in the future, but I can say from my experience people who know you will hang on every word if you take the time to record what happens. A journal can be in very simple chronological form with no concern about grammar or punctuation. Some of the things Renewal members shared with me were more like stream of consciousness writing. It was as if once they started to write, their words triggered an avalanche and they didn't know how to stop.

When my wife was treated for breast cancer she was conscientious about making her journal entries. She said she could vent about her illness and treatments in writing as a substitute for yelling at the medical staff.

Years ago a man named Ira Progoff, Ph.D., taught a traveling seminar on journal keeping. I attended and liked his approach. In essence Dr. Progoff recommended a loose leaf notebook with tabs inserted for every category of your life: job, spouse, children, parents, illness—everything. He felt that entries would vary in their emphasis day to day. With his method different subjects could be kept organized chronologically and easy to refer to. That way over time you can look back at any category and follow how your perceptions of that subject changed.

—⁂—

A variation on journaling is to use what you write to search for hidden meanings. Someone once observed that there is nothing in our future that is not already in our consciousness. If you can accept that, then the task is how to penetrate and get perspective on your total consciousness. This is probably at the limit of what a new student should undertake, but it is safe and worth your trying. To begin put yourself in a relaxed situation and start writing whatever comes to mind. Use the hand you normally write with. Pose what you write in the form of a question. Direct it to some part of your physical body, maybe your cancer if you have one. Query your mind asking if there are worries needing to surface. Then, use your non-dominant hand to write the answer. It is better to have different colored pens in each hand to accentuate separation. Do not try to modify, clarify, or correct the spontaneity of whatever words show up on the paper. If you have a trusted friend or advisor, discuss what your Q&A comments might mean.

This exercise is based upon the idea that one side of the brain usually dominates and is associated with your intellect. This side, usually the left, is constantly analyzing, constantly processing, constantly synthesizing to keep itself busy. It is accustomed to being in control, making decisions and telling you what to do. The other, non-dominant side of your brain is just as active, but doesn't speak up in your normal activities. The latter is your creative, intuitive side. According to convention it is the part of you where new ideas are created. These creative insights are just as much a part of you, but quiet like a child who is happily playing alone.

Your dominant brain tells you what to do; the non-dominant self plays on until you ask it something. The latter is content because it is not buried in the drudgery of everyday problems of existence. It will assist you with fresh ideas in many predicaments. Writing with the non-dominant hand is a straightforward way to gain access to new information. For several billion years no one was on earth to enjoy sunsets or see rainbows. Does that mean they did not exist? Our non-dominant brain is like that; it is neutral about revealing itself. We have to go to it and ask.

Drawing pictures of illness and perceptions is a similar exercise in self-inquiry. I still remember participating in a workshop with a large group of executives years ago. One assignment was drawing pictures of how we saw ourselves in life. The person in charge said draw ourselves somewhere at home with as much detail as possible. When everyone had finished we went around the room and held up our drawing to explain it. One very bright woman executive did as she was told. She held up a detailed picture of her living room and stood up to explain its contents. Here was the couch with a special fabric, here some chairs, there the mantle and fireplace with logs burning, assorted pictures on the walls. Even her cat was drawn in. As she spoke I, like everyone else, began to lean forward searching for what we did not see. The facilitator finally posed our question for us, "And where are you in this picture?"

"Oh," the woman said, surprised we didn't get it. She pointed to eight tiny bumps along the bottom margin of her picture, "here I am. That's my fingers on the handlebars. I'm riding my exercycle!" If you draw your self, you are the central part of the exercise; don't relegate yourself to insignificance.

Using art can be expressive and revealing of inner truth, but requires careful analysis and interpretation. This may not be a good place for you to start unless you have access to someone experienced in this work, but there is some introduction to this in Nancy and Bill's story in Chapter 3.

You are in a mode of learning and doing and you expect results. Being judgmental causes static. Learning comes quickest when you play. New research shows the whole brain lights up when presented with a new activity or challenge. Conversely, brain activity slows when doing the same old things over and over. Doing something, whether it be journal writing or imagery, or anything else new, you will make mistakes. You are not stupid; you just don't know how to do this new activity yet. You need practice so go ahead and begin.

Moving along, consider developing a set of personal rituals or ceremonies you can relate to. You do not need a lot of formal instruction to get started. Some people get this as part of their religion. However you feel about religion, create something private and unique to your own life. This can begin with items you retained from school or military service. Maybe something you found on a hike or a ceremony is important. Maybe it is a souvenir purchased at a special place during a trip abroad.

George W. (Chapter 3) once gave me a tie clasp. Misreading the situation, I protested that I shouldn't be accepting gifts. George corrected my thinking. He said this was a prized memento from his being in the Navy in WWII. He wanted me to have it. While I was turning the tie clasp over in my fingers and trying to think of what to say, George cleared up the matter in his characteristic gruff voice: "I want you to have it, Doc," he fixed his steely blue-eyed gaze upon me, "because I love you." I still have that tie clasp.

Maybe someone like a parent gave you a memento that has been in the family for generations. Maybe this is a time for you to pick something new that symbolizes your fight against cancer, something like an eagle or an owl. Is there some other creature or structure you associate with your struggle? If so, adopt it as your own.

Some people take a further step in this direction similar to what Native Americans once did. Do this by choosing an animal that you feel best symbolizes who you really are. This can draw upon anything from the brute strength of a buffalo or bear to the cunning and wiliness of a fox or coyote. Maybe you see yourself associating with a spirit more harmless like an otter, a rabbit, or a frog. Creating a private ritual around this idea gives you the opportunity to seek wisdom from such a partner while you renew your self.

Anything like this can start strengthening your association with a new reality. It becomes the talisman of what you will become. The advantage is, such a process can be completely private. It does not have to be shared with anyone, at least until you feel ready to share. A famous European psychiatrist once observed that the most valuable thing a person possesses is the secrets they know. A personal ritual you create can be part of your new power and is yours alone.

Others look for spiritual guides and contacts with beings beyond what we can see, but that is beyond the scope of this book. I will mention that my wife has high regard for both her maternal grandmother and one maternal aunt. Both of these women had great influence when my wife was growing up. Both have been dead for years. Anytime my wife needs a quick bit of help, whether it be finding a convenient parking spot when out shopping, or seeking a better seat on a crowded airplane, she calls upon one of these two relatives for help. As far as I know, one or the other has always furnished the assistance requested.

Try starting in the morning asking, "What can I do today that will bring happiness into my life? What can I do for fun?" If you make your answer the top priority for each day, many of us feel you will have taken one of the most important steps possible in regaining your sense of well being. We all know people who died during times of duress. By comparison, how many people have you heard of who died while having a great time? And if someone does die in a joyous moment, how do you feel about that?

Daniel L. Reardon said, "In the long run the pessimist may be proved right, but the optimist has a better time on the trip."

Renewal is not anti-intellectual; it just recognizes that you cannot think your way back to health. Action is necessary. New experiences actually cause DNA in our brain to synthesize new proteins to store that memory. Our actions modify our brain. Part of that action is to educate your self. The search for your ideal diet, strengthening the immune system and use of supplements are just three reasons to do research on your own. There are countless books to help you. As soon as you find something that makes sense, act upon it. Become proactive and curious. A recent report indicates that in a given year one quarter of our population does not read a single book and that's discouraging. Still, reading and educating your self will fortify you to question authority.

Strive for mental health. Look to eliminate harmful influences and unnecessary stress in your life. Confront relationships draining your energy. Try to minimize TV and reading newspapers for a time to see if this helps.

Whenever you feel tired, rest. A relaxed mind is creative and less likely to make mistakes.

Some suggestions about diet and exercise are in Appendices II and III. The present chapter is about the more global problem of how to overcome apathy and paralysis of fear. Have you ever heard the question, "Which is worse, ignorance or apathy?" And the response, "I don't know and I don't care!" Don't let this be you.

Most of us can recognize our self talk about who we are. When we get a serious illness like cancer that self talk says something like, "This is not right!" Or, "I don't deserve this!" Another person says to themselves, "I'm old and useless. Maybe this cancer is my quick ticket out of here!" Maybe you do feel you have overstayed and it is time to go. In any event cancer will invalidate some of your options. We suggest canceling these negative thoughts. Create a set of affirmations that give your subconscious a clear set of positive directions. Re-read the section about the Pacific Institute's approach. Zig Ziglar said, "Positive thinking will let you do everything better than negative thinking will."

It's OK to gather statistics and ask your physicians about prognosis and—just don't accept uncritically everything you are told. Most people with serious illness have longer than they think. What if you have another five or ten years, or even longer? How do you know you don't? "Because my doctor says so," is not an acceptable answer. For the moment can we just agree that you are here? If you can accept there is some reason you are still alive, some purpose, then you have turned to face in the correct direction. You are ready to start your journey.

The people in Renewal started where you are right now. They had nothing more to work with than you have. Some of them achieved extraordinary results. They began with the simple premises about reason and purpose given to them in our meetings. Illness was the starting point of their renewal. On the whole, members of Renewal were successful. The successful ones found in his or her own way a meaning for life and extended themselves. They did the necessary work. Remember Artie in Chapter 2? She had five separate cancers treated before she died—all of them serious. Every time some new challenge turned up she faced it with determination and good humor. Several other stories in this book are about people with not just cancer but also another debilitating illness adding to their burden.

What follows is not meant to confuse you or dilute our central message, but I believe you will benefit from thinking more deeply about where your ideas and assumptions come from. My hope is that when you understand that many things you accept do not have deep roots, you may be more willing to pull them out. You can choose to replace them with new ideas that serve you better.

The way medicine is practiced in the United States is based upon a model that is only a little over a hundred years old. It was based upon the discovery of micro-organisms and a subsequent formulation of how much of disease is caused by bacteria, viruses, and parasites. It was only a hundred years ago that the Flexner Report led to a reorganization of how medical schools would teach based only upon the scientific method.

You may think you aren't interested in how things were done back then. Where you should see relevance is to hear that less than half the medical treatments in common use today have a scientific basis, i.e., objectively have been proven to work. On the patient side, complaints leading to more than half of all office and ER visits are not found to have any organic basis. A physician friend who works full time in a hospital emergency room calls his shift "The Granny Clinic." In effect he says if most patients had a grandmother at home to ask for advice (about treating bee stings, rashes, problems with breast feeding, and the like) they would never be in the emergency department waiting for hours to be seen. Few people realize that many drugs they take and the treatments they receive have not been shown either to prolong or improve the quality of life. Many popular screening tests for cancer cannot be shown to increase cure rates or prolong life. So if you hear that a malignancy responds to chemotherapy or radiation, be sure to follow up with a question to your physician: ask what that specifically means to you.

Much of surgery is based upon only the assumption that doing an operation is good and will benefit the patient, not upon proof. Twenty years ago tonsillectomies were one of the most common operations performed in the United States. When they were shown not to result in any benefit, the profession mostly stopped doing them. Much the same is true about performing hysterectomies. When I was trained and went into practice there was a complicated system of operations on the stomach for peptic ulcers. It was built around acceptance that ulcer disease was caused by excess acid. When a bacterial cause for most ulcers was discovered about 20 years ago, our whole approach to stomach surgery became passé. The same is true about the flourishing drug industry for treating elevated cholesterol levels. Many Americans don't need this treatment and never will see any benefit from it. It is almost the same for operations for coronary bypass and stent placement that benefit so few. If you doubt this, ask your own physician what the evidence is either for prevention or increasing longevity with these treatment modalities compared to lifestyle changes alone.

I spent most of my career in a conventional surgical practice. This is not meant to be a diatribe against allopathic medicine. Many treatments produce good results but many others do not. Part of your job is to gather pertinent answers. Sift through what you are told about treatments and decide which are likely to work and which are not. Ask questions. It is your body, your therapy. You are paying for treatment on many levels, not just the economic one. Most of the members of Renewal felt they benefited from their care but learned to be cautious in accepting medical advice. These opinions of mine are meant to stimulate your thinking about cancer treatment as various options are presented to you.

Accepting medical care is a leap of faith, especially when treatment is expensive and/or toxic. We as physicians never know if a medicine or operation will help an individual. We have to rely upon best evidence and law of averages.

The decisions you make can have a great deal to do with outcome—for cure and for quality of life. One thing to emphasize again, shown in the Renewal experience, is how much you can do for your self when properly informed and empowered by your own resolve. Since complementary treatments and self help are unlikely to do any harm, I believe they can be held to a different standard. Much of the information about supplements has been anecdotal but that is beginning to change. Witness the current interest in Vitamin D in preventing several cancers. Recent reports suggest it even may prevent many cases of Type I diabetes. With these last comments in mind, go back and re-read the approach presented by Dr. Jonathan Collin in Chapter 7. Another source of new ideas and contrarian opinion is a newsletter published by Julian Whitaker MD: www.drwhitaker.com.

The relevance for you is how much medicine is changing. It will continue to evolve. Robotic surgery has come to mean patient and surgeon do not have to be in the same room or even on the same continent. Random drug trials remove a lot of discretion from the hands of the treating physician. Attempts to amass personal medical records in databanks of Google and Microsoft will reframe discussions about privacy and personal information. The federal program called the Health Insurance Portability and Accountability Act (HIPAA) has ironically destroyed both privacy and any common-sense transmission of health information. How much of this is good, and where it will all end up, I don't know.

This is worth reviewing because all these are examples of mental models. A man named Kenneth J. Gergen put forth in his writing, "Research findings don't have any meaning until they are interpreted...They result from a process of negotiating meaning within a community..." When information gets to the level of treating physician and cancer patient, we share it as if it is reality. It may be true and maybe not.

If we study acupuncture we find that its energy points and flow make no allowance for the concept most westerners see as established facts concerning anatomy and the nervous system. Anyone who has ever studied anatomy will tell you they can clearly identify our peripheral nervous system. They know how nerves connect to our brain. They know there is a micro-environment surrounding individual nerves where chemical reactions occur and generate electrical impulses. They know this on both a cellular and molecular level.

Acupuncture is taught in Asia and throughout the world without inclusion of what Western allopathic medicine identifies as the filamentous structures we call nerves. For acupuncture practitioners it is all energy and flow. It has nothing to do with anatomy as we describe it. A physician friend of mine who is an expert in acupuncture says that the concept of energy flow, the Qi, or chi, is non-corporeal. It simply has no correlation to conventional Western medicine but it works. One system is actual and we see it, one is virtual. Acupuncture is an art. It also has a science that works for whole societies. It simply is supported by a different set of facts in a different community of practitioners.

For hundreds of years physicians were taught an art of medical practice that did not recognize what our circulatory system does. Physicians of old knew there was a heart and ascribed to it attributes like love and valor. They knew there was blood. Blood was accepted as one of the primary humors of the body. They also saw there were tubes throughout the body containing blood. They did not recognize this tied together as an essential function, conduits carrying a fluid circulating nutrients and removing metabolic wastes.

Even if we restrict ourselves to the field of current medical thought we can see how it becomes essential for practitioners and patients to share beliefs. Both physician and patient are in the habit of recruiting others to share their model of reality. We learn to screen for information that conforms to our mental model of illness. If you are not accepting my set of medical "facts," you and I do not have anything to build a conversation upon. People become emotional, even frantic, to convince you to accept their reality. Because beliefs are nothing more than a perceived model of what exists, the implication is you are attempting to invalidate my reality if you do not share it. If you are not accepting, you move outside my thinking and become other. Conflict may ensue.

For our purposes here, the medical model you have, and your concept of illness, only exists between you and anyone else who shares that belief with you. You reach an agreement and thus form a basis for action. This becomes possible because we are communicating through the same language. We use the same sounds as "words" to name the physical world and its actions. It's the same way we accept current hypotheses of quantum mechanics explaining esoteric parts of physics, mostly because we (and nobody else) understand them. Treatises on quantum mechanics explain some of what is observed about the universe, but not everything.

The relevance to our story about Renewal is that medical science is constructed in the same way. This is why having a group of people like Renewal to relate to can be important in rebuilding health. What you believe to be true about medicine as a discipline (even worse, self-talk telling yourself you are too ignorant to make decisions and are not capable of understanding technical information) may lead you to accept some doctrinaire statements in your course of treatment. Same is true of assertions or assumptions about why you became ill. What you are told may be right. It may be wrong. Confusion about the validity of facts and truth may cause you to disregard intuition and your own capabilities. You may decide to cede decisions about your well-being to others.

Your future life may depend upon who makes your decisions. Will it be you or someone else? Which way do you feel this balance tips? Is it shifting to your advantage or in another way? You may accept, in a similar manner, conclusions about your prognosis. Most of the things we deal with in life are ephemeral and many illusionary. Constants are few. We have a concept of who we are and what we need. We sustain this physical body of ours by supplying it with shelter, water, food, and a few other essentials. There are things (money, citizenship, possibly the concept of health) that exist only because we accept they exist. The fear is that my body, my self, is at a disadvantage. I have no durability. If we allow ourselves to think about death, we fear it. Dying is so counter to the interests of a healthy mind that we cannot process the concept of going out of existence. What we see in the graph below on the left side is how most people see life stacked up in terms of relative importance.

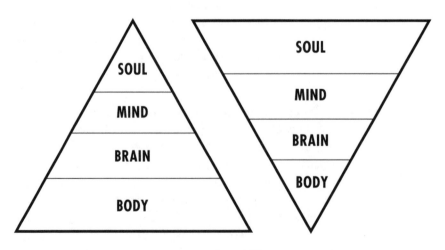

Most people consider their physical body most important as represented proportionately on the left.
An alternative concept is to the right.

Most of us will accept that our body is directed in its functions by the brain. We will say that even if we have never seen any part of the nervous system. We may know that even the hormones secreted from our endocrine glands are under the direction of a master gland at the base of the brain. That master gland is stimulated by connections to the central nervous system. The brain worries, it has ideas. One outcome of research is the suggestion that the collection of nerve cells in the brain is very good at telling stories. What the mind does is less clear. The mind is offered up in this book as a practical ally to use in trying to regain or maintain our health. Soul is even more remote in our deliberations. Since we cannot dissect it out of the body, does it even exist? If you believe you have a soul, does it too cease to exist at the moment we die, as we think the conscious mind does?

Whether you are interested or not, this awareness of brain function and of consciousness leads to the conclusion that reality, what we see around us, is nothing more, nothing less, than something we created within our individual brains. Some of this is oral traditions, songs, legends, myths, objects of worship, things we differentiate in our thinking and make acceptable. Some of the things we do in Renewal bring back those rituals, especially reviving Native American traditions, allowing us to tap into more primitive beliefs. We at once avoid the polemics that might arise if we choose to use the language of a particular Christian sect or other religion. In so doing we introduce non-threatening ways of thinking that our minds are willing to accept.

The meditations in Appendix I are a modification of storytelling. Try using them. The ideal would be to have a trusted friend read the meditations to you. Get into a relaxed atmosphere first then see if you can begin to appreciate what your mind will do for you if you speak to it in a language it understands. Perhaps we can agree that these concepts can become the map—our mental map—that allows our inner self to refute harmful old beliefs. Replacing our old map is a first step in laying out our healing process differently. It lets us begin anew.

Ancient mystics taught a concept of soul and mind generating our physical bodies. Such a message has been tumultuous but consistent through the ages. What if The Creator did in fact project an initial pulse of energy to create and vivify everything we know? Maybe it would be better to focus our energy on ascending the triangle on the right. *(See image on previous page.)* That is, pay less attention to the body and try to reconnect to the soul. The implication implies something difficult, i.e., the scaling of an overhang. Here rising to each new level of abstraction introduces a broader spectrum than the level below it. Such an effort of personal growth, novel as it may prove to be, has potential to become more rewarding than investigating only functions of the physical body (the left side).

What's the purpose of taking a sojourn into something as philosophical as the last few pages? One person who sums this up well is Lama Zopa Rinpoche in his book, *Ultimate Healing* (Wisdom Publications, Boston, 2001): "Everything comes from the mind…Chinese medical texts explain that all diseases originate in the mind and relate sickness to the three fundamental delusions: ignorance, anger, and attachment…we have to heal the causes of suffering, which are in our mental continuum. The way any object appears to us…depends…upon how we label it. It is clear that it is our own concept that is experiencing disease. First our mind labels something, then we see it." And he goes on to quote another yogi, Naropa, who said, "When we are sick, the concept is sick."

With this idea in mind, let your thinking return to the people you read about in Chapters 2 and 3. Think of the approaches group members used in personal renewal. Think of the outcomes they had. Compare to assumptions and expectations about your own illness. Consider putting some of Renewal's ideas to use. The people and the continuing spirit of the Renewal cancer support group wish you well. With new resolve read the suggestions for action steps in the Appendices that follow.

I believe this book has given what is needed to start your new path. Before we conclude, here is one more concept of renewal for you. Add this to the others for creating the broadest perspective. It is a finishing component as you move forward to your own way of healing. From the Thanksgiving Psalms in the Dead Sea Scrolls comes the statement, "Life always begins again." And Kabir (1398-1518?) wrote in his Sakhi Sangrah:

What I was once,
I am not now.
I have reaped the benefit
Of my precious human birth;

APPENDICES

APPENDIX I
MEDITATIONS

Here are three meditations written by Renewal member Nancy K., whose personal story about inflammatory breast cancer appears in Chapter 2. Nancy provided these exercises for the book based upon her personal healing and the work she continues with others. Ideally you can record these or have someone take you through each one by reading aloud. For now, just read each one to your self. Experience what they are designed to do.

— Health Meditation —

Find an appropriate space where you will not be disturbed for a while. You can sit in a comfy chair or lie down, whichever you prefer. Put your body in a comfortable position with your hands resting in your lap. Take a deep, slow breath and gently close your eyes. As you breathe in through your nose become aware of your inhale, allowing it to fill and expand your abdomen just below the waistline. Hold the breath for a comfortable amount of time then exhale gently through your mouth. Continue to breathe this deeply, counting each breath until you reach ten. Return to normal calm breathing. Now you find yourself relaxed and at peace. Your body feels content, warm and safe. Your mind is at ease.

As you become accustomed to this gentle feeling you see in your mind's eye a stream. The stream is flowing gently between plush banks covered with ferns and grasses. The water runs over rocks and into crevices making a lovely babbling sound. This is so pleasant that you begin to walk along the bank. The further you go the more clearly you hear the sound of water. It sounds louder with each step you take. As you look ahead you see a waterfall. It is not big, just barely taller than you are. The water looks so inviting that you reach out your hand and touch it. It is warm and soft and falls on a flat rock platform, barely splashing when it hits. Knowing that you are safe and secure you step out onto the flat rock platform and let the water fall on your body. It feels so good. You realize that this is a magical place. The water is there to help you heal. It can heal any disease, any stress, and all concerns that you may have. While the water flows over your head and down around you, tranquility fills every cell of your body.

While you are enjoying this feeling the water begins to turn red. This ruby color gives you energy and life. Each and every cell soaks up the experience. Then the water begins to turn orange. It brings you oxygen to revive cell growth and energize your immune system. You can feel these effects instantly taking place inside of you. Now the water changes to yellow. The yellow water brings with it an increase in your strength, long-lasting, ever-present strength. When your body wills itself, with all that it needs of this strength, the water adjusts to green. This is the color of health; each cell that needs attention takes the healthy gifts from the green water. Any disease that might be present is washed away with each drop. Revel in this water; it is here to serve you. When you're ready, the water changes to blue, a clear, perfect blue. As the blue runs over your body you are given peace; emotional peace, mental peace and physical peace. All of the systems in your body now work together, harmoniously, for the greater good of your life. As this feeling of calm becomes familiar to you the water switches to purple. The violet water blesses you with a sense of self worth. You realize that you have every right to be alive, to be healthy, and to be strong. You accept your birthright, knowing that this is so. As you are invigorated by this understanding the water becomes silvery white and transparent. You are refreshed, renewed, revitalized and healed.

As you step out from under the waterfall you know that you can return. You may return here any time that you doubt, even for a second, that you are the wonderful, strong, alive, being that you see right now. This is your inheritance, this is you life.

Knowing that every cell in your body is responding to the gifts that you have just given it, you know that it is time to come back. Become aware again of where you are. Feel the way your body is reclining. Feel the breath as it fills you with oxygen to carry on with all that is your life. Move slightly to feel your fingers and toes. Whenever you are ready you can open your eyes.

— Relaxation Meditation —

Sit in a comfortable position, hands gently lying in your lap. Take a slow, deep breath and close your eyes. Allow your mouth to drop open slightly to relax your jaw. Bring your attention to your breath. Slowly inhale and count to four; hold the breath to four beats then slowly exhale while counting to four. Continue this pattern and feel your body relax with each exhale. Feel yourself sinking into the chair, snuggling into blissful comfort. You feel safe and warm and secure.

As you continue to relax and sink, your breath returns to normal. Now, you see before you a path. This path wanders through a sunlit field of wildflowers. There are small yellow daisies and tiny white snowdrops, in between them are rivers of bright blue bachelor's buttons. The small dirt path beckons you to walk along it. As you begin to stroll along you see a forest before you. The forest abounds with inviting trees and greenery. You can see shafts of sunlight falling between the tall straight trees. The closer you get the more you can feel the cool dampness of the forest air. It looks and feels like the most welcoming place you have ever encountered.

As you enter the forest, the path becomes carpeted with pine needles and fern fronds. Each step is cushioned with these offerings from the environment. You feel surrounded by safety and familiarity. All apprehension, anxiety and stress from your day are relieved with each step that you take. The forest is enveloping you with comfort.

As you go further into the thick of the trees, the light dims yet you can still see easily. You are overcome with a gentle feeling of finally being home. In front of you is a stone bench. As you sit down on the bench you know that all that may have bothered you in your life today is being gently and deliberately cleared away by the joy that flows to you in your perfect spot amongst these giant living trees. The oxygen, lovingly given to you by nature, is restoring your body, enlivening your mind and enriching your spirit. Sit here for as long as you wish. Allow yourself to be unwound and separated from the day, tranquilized from the stress, and calmed past any tensions. Know that you can come back to this place and these same feelings any time that you want. You only have to take a few minutes, close your eyes, breathe and walk down this little path.

Now it is time to return, refreshed and revitalized. Whenever you are ready, take a deep breath and become aware of your body and its position. Become aware of your surroundings and slowly and easily open your eyes.

— Cancer Meditation —

I did this meditation every night when I first went to bed. It helped me calm my mind from all the frightening thoughts that swirled around when the house was dark and quiet. I was able to let go of the feeling that the disease controlled my life. I also used this every day that I had chemo. After all the tubes were in and running I had several hours while the infusion process went on. I would snuggle in the recliner as best I could, wrap a heated blanket around me, and try to relax. This is what I used to kill the beast that was threatening me. -Nancy K.

Find a safe spot, away from any distractions or interruptions. Sit in a cozy chair or lie down if you prefer, and close your eyes. Put your hands in a comfortable position by your side or in your lap. Take a slow, deep breath. Hold it for a second then slowly exhale. Feel yourself being surrounded by a fluffy, warm blanket. Nestle into it. Feel the safety and calm of this space. Continue to breathe slowly, concentrating on your breath until you can feel yourself sinking and relaxing. Release all the tension from your muscles, become aware of their becoming heavy, peaceful, and at rest. Release the tension from your bones. Know that they are letting go of all the stresses of your disease and its treatment.

As you settle in to the pleasant, restful sensations that are enveloping your body, see in your mind's eye a large screen, like the ones in movie theatres. You find yourself easily sitting in front of it. Slowly the screen becomes bright and you can see yourself illuminated on it. As you look at your body projected before you, you realize that you can control and manipulate the picture. Look carefully at your body. Ask to see the disease. The areas where the disease is located become dark and are well defined. Find the spot on your body where the disease is closest to the skin. You can see it clearly.

In your mind's eye, stand up and walk to the screen. Reach out and touch that spot. When you can feel it, reach inside your image and feel the end of a rope. Without hesitation you know that rope is attached to the cancer. Now it's your turn to take control of it: begin to pull. The rope is black and slimy but slides out easily. Each cancer cell that is affecting your health comes out as a knot along the rope. Continue to pull on the rope and knots as long as it takes to get to the end. Cancer cells are weak; there are just a lot of them doing their dirty work. You can see that the dark spot on your skin is much lighter and clearer now. Look again: see if there is another spot that needs your attention. If so, go to it and pull out that rope and knots.

When you are satisfied that you have cleared all the areas of cancer, or have done all you can today, return to your seat. Look at the image on the screen. You look so much better, more healthy, energized, and alive. You realize, too, that you feel much lighter and it is easier to breathe. Now that your work is done for the moment, relax into the comfort of this warm, safe spot that your physical body is in right now.

Remember whenever cancer becomes scary or you become fearful for any reason, you can come back to this place, this method, of healing. Here you are in control. Cancer can be cast out like garbage. Whenever you are ready, become aware of your body and its position in the chair. Slowly wiggle your fingers and toes, feeling them move and flex. Stretch your arms and legs and open your eyes.

APPENDIX II
DIET

This is not going to be a summary list of things to do. I don't think such lists are taken seriously or influence behavior much. Besides, I don't like lists and I don't like people telling me what to do. You may feel the same way. So I am going to reason with you a bit and make this brief. I hope if this is short enough, and you've gotten this far in the book, you will not be able to resist reviewing this call to action.

Quick sermon: with all the worry about cancer you would think people would pay attention to the fact so many cancers can be prevented. According to our federal government at least two-thirds of cancers are preventable. Many scientists put that figure even higher. The total breaks down to one-third if everyone quit smoking (most lung cancers, but also mouth and esophagus). Another third is caused by diet aberrations. Only 5-10% of cancers are caused by single inherited genes and an estimated 1% by industrial chemicals. These prevention numbers become impressive when applied to a particular malignancy: a high fiber diet, supplemental vitamin D, and periodic colonoscopy take care of most colon cancer. We also enter a dichotomy: Is the reader's interest prevention of cancer or adjuncts to cure disease you already have? But let's press on...

Comprehending all the factors involving cancer is huge and gets hazy at the edges. On a worldwide scale, sweeping generalizations become more complicated. In some countries infection may be responsible for up to one-fourth of all cancers. Findings and "facts" are all over the place and make dogmatic assertions difficult. Fortunately more information becomes available all the time to clarify what is true. Most cancers require several steps to initiate growth. Such new growths, or neoplasms, occur because of influences on genetic material that take years or even decades to manifest themselves. The more one studies data the easier it is to accept that a healthy existence has us in a state of balance. Some substances and activities in our cells promote abnormal growth. Other cellular processes inhibit deviations or provide surveillance protecting us. We also have an elegant system of immunity (lymphocytes, antibodies, cytokines and the like) to deal with cancer at the cellular level.

We have all read numbers about how many cells we have in our body or how many in our brain. More important is the estimate that over an average lifetime your body's cells will have 10^{16} (ten with sixteen zeroes after it) divisions. Each division is an opportunity for something to go wrong. Any wrong step conceivably can induce a cancer. Not only that, it is estimated that 95% of the cells in your body are microbes. Viruses perpetuate themselves by diverting intracellular machinery to enhance their own survival. A virologist I knew once told me human beings are little more than walking bags of viruses. Other scientists cynically observe humans may only exist as vectors for a higher purpose of propagating viruses.

Something must go right since we humans have survived so far, even though it is a complex matter. The 25,000 or more bioactive components in the average human diet play a huge role. We cannot influence cellular chemistry with our intellect (at least most of us don't think we can) but we can make intelligent choices about what we eat and what to avoid. Enough data exists where we all should be able to make good decisions about what to eat. Much of the data presented here is extracted from the recent report "Food, Nutrition, Physical Activity, and the Prevention of Cancer" compiled by the World Cancer Research Fund and American Institute for Cancer Research. Copies are available by contacting them at 1759 R Street NW, Washington DC 20009.

Their report published in 2007 brought together all the objective data from the previous five years and evaluated it for veracity and relevance. The report is about 500 pages long, quite detailed but largely understandable and cohesive. I recommend you obtain a copy and study it if you are serious about advancing your knowledge. The report boils down to eight primary recommendations with two additions:

1. Be as lean as possible within the normal range of body weight. Ab-

dominal fatness is associated with most cancers.
2. Be physically active as part of everyday life.
3. Limit energy-dense foods and avoid sugary drinks.
4. Eat mostly foods of plant origin.
5. Limit intake of red meat; avoid processed meat.
6. Limit alcoholic drinks. Alcohol is associated with risk for most cancers.
7. Limit consumption of salt; avoid moldy cereal grains and legumes.
8. Aim to meet nutritional needs through diet alone. This report does not recommend supplements for cancer prevention.
9. A special recommendation is added for cancer survivors to follow all the recommendations for prevention.
10. And for anyone who would be affected, breast feeding is recommended exclusively for the first six months of an infant's life.

The unifying concept bringing components of this 2007 report together is a combination of strengthening your immune system plus stress reduction. In this book about Renewal every few pages something appears about positive-thinking, canceling negative thoughts, and reducing stress. We have been conditioning your thinking. I hope you realize that and now it is time for you to take over.

The immune system is the surveillance and combat force. Your role is to supply your defenses with what they need to win the struggle. This is basically the food you ingest plus avoiding harmful substances like alcohol, pesticides, etc. If you do these things, you will have done your part. Study of the immune system is complex. The average reader does not know much about immunology, or biochemistry, or physiology. Fortunately you don't have to.

As Kimberly Mathai recommended in Chapter 7, eat your vegetables and fruit with attention to getting the widest possible variety of color. The molecules signified by those colors will be attracted to where to go to do their job. Take a multivitamin with extra vitamin C. It is now evident that taking higher doses of Vitamin D is important, at least 1000-2000 units per day. Be sure to get zinc and selenium. Conversely, most people with cancer do not need supplemental iron.

The variations on diet and supplements are almost endless. There are plenty of other things to consider like detoxification, cleansing diets and fasting. For years I avoided eating on Mondays. I felt this was a way to cut food consumption, remind myself of health discipline, and focus attention on beginning a new week. This idea, like so much of what we all do, had value because I believed in what I was doing. After a time I moved away from that regimen. I don't think there has been a month in the last 30 years I haven't changed some part of what I do to be healthy. You will probably make such modifications too; it's OK.

I do not recommend you do anything outside conventional recommendations unless you do your own investigation and it makes sense to you. This is really the secret behind many self-help initiatives. It is the essence of why we need to get clear on our purpose and focus before we start. Then, be eclectic in choosing sources of information to act upon. Go slow in making new commitments. In general moderation is the best course, at least until you have gathered sufficient information to do otherwise.

Though I wish everyone would do their own investigation, there are a number of reasons why we don't. I am going to give you a nudge in the right direction by telling you what I do most of the time, based upon nearly 40 years of looking. My purpose is to let you know how simple getting started can be: Each morning I get a head start with a 12 ounce serving of low sodium V8 juice. I buy it by the case. To this juice I add several dashes of ground cayenne red pepper and a scoop of D-ribose powder. The latter is for the ATP-ADP cycle, our energy source for most intracellular metabolism. The component in this chemical reaction most likely to be deficient is the sugar D-ribose. It is not a cheap supplement but is readily available.

While I am doing that my wife uses our blender to make a health drink: whey or soy protein powder, frozen berries, ground flax seed, banana, skim milk, and resveratrol tonic (an anti-oxidant—we currently use one from LifeTime, www.lifetimevitamins.com). That plus several cups of good hot tea—Maureen is Irish—washes down a small handful of vitamins. Choosing supplements is the kind of thing you can do for yourself.

I advocate doing this first when you get up and after that, getting dressed for the day. I was fortunate in medical school to have studied under the foremost physiologist of the 20th century, Dr. Arthur C. Guyton. Among many things I remember he advocated to our class: First, a hot drink or hot food at breakfast time. That warmth initiates the gastro-colic reflex. A normal intestinal tract will be stimulated to empty itself, a very healthy process, but you have to give it 10-15 minutes to do so. That won't happen if you skip breakfast or eat going out the door. Getting up earlier is the solution to creating the extra time. Rising early allows a few moments to read, meditate, or "prosecute" the coming day as Benjamin Franklin once advised. Fluids plus these extra few minutes potentiate the bulk (fiber) you have in your diet and promote bowel regularity.

Second, Dr. Guyton told us the physiologist he respected most ate only one egg a year. "He said he ate one just so he wouldn't forget what they taste like," Dr. Guyton said with a smile. He was too wise to tell even compliant medical students what to do and left it up to us to deduce why a wise person might not eat eggs.

The morning routine I described, including the cup of berries, provides six of the recommended daily servings of fruit and vegetables along with half of the protein. At noon eat what you want, but let it include low fat protein. Protein at mid-day helps avoid energy drop in the afternoon. The evening meal I consider a bonus meal since I have already had everything I consider obligatory. Other ideas like five small meals a day, bedtime snacks, are all worth considering as you individualize and create your own approach. There are many plans for you to choose from, especially if you work with a dietician. The example I made about my diet at home just handles most of the nutrition issue for a whole day at breakfast time. After breakfast I can coast. I am getting older now and like to enjoy everything I do. Like me, try not to let the whole issue of food, which should be one of life's pleasures, cause stress.

By the way, while I'm dispensing advice, be careful where you get information. On television the day before I wrote this, a reporter interviewed a local chef about goodies he was preparing for our upcoming County Fair. The woman reporter picked up one non-descript item on the table and asked, "This is your famous fried Spam, isn't it?" The rather rotund chef nodded well, yes, it was. "This is low fat, isn't it?" the reporter asked ambiguously, tearing a crisp brown piece of battered Spam apart with her fingers.

"Yes," the chef said, nodding his agreement, "We fry the fat right out of it!"

Here's one suggestion for the evening meal, especially if you have access to a market that carries prepackaged mixes of greens such as spinach, collard, mustard, all washed and cut. Recipes are on the package. It is very easy to cook greens on the stove top with a cup of vegetable broth and/or tomato juice. Add a can of chopped tomatoes and chilies or white beans, or both, and you have another tasty vegetable dish. This has low energy density, or fewer calories per unit volume, and fills you up as a whole meal. It supplies the green leafy vegetables many cooks don't know how to prepare and is just the kind of creative thing you want with your vegetable selections.

And as Ms. Mathai wrote in Chapter 7, let the system make life easier for you. One package of these greens should provide enough servings for several meals. All you have to do is put leftovers in the refrigerator and reheat when you want. Many recipes allow you to prepare several meals at once. Kimberly suggests some guidelines about serving size: half a cup of vegetables is one serving, a tennis ball equals one cup, and something the size of a computer mouse is about three ounces.

Frances Moore Lappe's book, *Diet for a Small Planet* (1971), is an educational classic in this field. But you don't need it or anything else as a new bible in order to start replacing the energy-dense meat and white stuff on your plate. Getting started is the key. Try to become good or excellent at this, not achieve perfection. A recent Harvard study indicated that if you think nine servings of vegetables and fruit a day is impossible, even five will be an excellent start. It's like sunscreen; SPF 30 is not noticeably more effective than SPF 15. The important thing is to participate, <u>do something.</u>

Look, I grew up around some people who have never—ever!—eaten a vegetable other than potatoes. For them it's meat, eggs, and maybe baked beans occasionally. And no salad either. I've got someone in my family who will excuse himself and leave the table if you put down a dish containing tofu. So I know there is resistance out there but I'm telling you, "Real evidence indicates things written here work and prevent cancer. Do you want to help your self or not?"

Here are a few more suggestions: Migrate gradually to the diet Kimberly Mathai recommends. As I've said, start to crowd the meat and starches off your plate by substituting any vegetables you like. Do you know strict vegetarians get cancer less often? What is the message there? Eating vegetables and fruit gives your body the alkaline or "sweet" nutrients it needs to maintain proper balance. Meat and just about anything animal-based adds to the acid or "sour" load on your system. Your body has to work extra hard to stay in balance when neutralizing excess acidity. Vegetables and plant-based foods maintain your system's alkalinity and that affects everything!

Make eating vegetables and fruit easy. Use pre-packaged and frozen products to start. If you are short on time, prepare food in larger quantity for multiple servings. Make a large pot of beans or lentils or brown rice or barley and serve out of that reserve for days. When you buy fresh produce, search for a farmer's market. Support the locals whenever you can. Try to choose organic as your sophistication grows. Take produce home and briefly soak in a sink of water with a couple of tablespoonfuls of Clorox added, then rinse. This kills off or oxidizes harmful residues that may have been in the soil or contaminated the supply chain. There are commercial rinses that do the same thing.

Obesity is a major factor associated with cancer. Increased abdominal girth increases risk of heart disease, premature death, and diabetes even when you are not overweight. This may be a problem for you and perhaps not. The quickest way to decide is to get a measuring tape right now. Measure your waist. Your circumference as a male should be 34 inches or less. If it is greater than 40 inches you have a real problem requiring attention. For women the comparable numbers are 27 inches or less with statistical evidence predicting trouble over 35 inches. This abdominal girth factor is directly related to consumption of sugar and the ubiquitous high fructose corn syrup hidden in so many prepared foods and drinks.

To maintain a healthy weight avoid eating in any of the fast food restaurants. Burgers and chicken prepared the fast food way are bad and super sizing is a terrible insult to digestion. Animal fats in general are unhealthy. Hydrogenated oils are unhealthy and a major component of most cookies and crackers and other things retailed in cardboard boxes. Read the labels!

Next is sugar intake. Sugar equates to empty calories. It causes derangement in the delicate balance of insulin supply and needed energy production. Sugar upsets our normal desire for good nutrition in much the same way alcoholic drinks do. An alcoholic can subsist on the ethanol they drink, but look at the outcome of that. Avoid drinking any kind of carbonated drinks like colas or juices with corn syrup. Anything that says fructose is posting a warning sign. Pure sugar harms your immune system, even if it is dissolved and hidden in a cola drink. Caution: the sugar substitutes used in diet drinks also are bad for you. They paradoxically increase your desire to eat. Research the subject of glycemic index so you will at least understand the principle involved.

Recall what Virginia Brown told Renewal about dealing with negative thoughts: when you have one, say "Cancel!" to yourself and substitute a positive image. The same principle can be applied to the food you ingest. This Appendix points out just a few things to get you started. Start reading and investigating on your own. Make the changes suggested if they make sense to you. Begin by choosing one area in your diet you are willing to change. Concentrate on that one thing. Delay adopting what you consider to be more draconian measures. Let change be gradual. Changing too much too fast may cause so much disruption in your system that backlash shocks you and you abandon the health initiative. You don't want that.

So in summary, see a healthy diet as an adjunct, the energy source for healing your self. Reduce your body's work load by supplying alkaline foods, vegetables and fruits. Eat colorful foods because the different colors are indicative of the presence of specific nutrients. Displace animal based foods and starches from your plate by adding more vegetables and fruit. If you are overweight, adopt a strategy for portion control. Avoid pure sugar, corn syrup or artificial sweeteners as much as possible. They compete with the innate desire to eat nutritious food and actually weaken your immune defense system. If you have never paid attention to nutrition before, don't know what to do, seek advice from a dietician interested in this subject. And after you have done one positive thing with your diet, do one with exercise.

APPENDIX III
EXERCISE

This section, like Appendix II on diet, is short in the hope you will read it. In the original plan for this book I assembled a large amount of information on physiology and all sorts of diagrams and figures to show specific stretches, weight-lifting forms, and yoga poses. I have put all that aside in order to say, the most important thing for you to do is move beyond intellectual knowing and *do something!*

Ralph Waldo Emerson once said we have to rise to a certain level of awareness before we can really take a walk. This book has placed heavy emphasis upon dealing with adversity by mental and spiritual preparedness to improve health. Hopefully now you feel prepared adequately to benefit from helping your self with another modality, exercise.

In the simplest form, your exercise program can be taking a walk. Even if you have cancer or are sick now from treatment it is likely your physician will OK an exercise program. If you have some physical disability that prevents walking, swimming, cycling or using a stationary apparatus may be better choices for you.

I keep this simple in the hope you will put on suitable shoes and go out and take a walk sometime in the next 24 hours. If you are physically or psychologically low right now, even this first step will have symbolic benefit: you can say you have started on an exercise program! Ideally you should have some advice from a professional trainer to judge your capability and map out a plan for progressing. A trainer will nudge you along and present variations to your program. The latter is important to avoid getting in a rut by using the same muscles all the time.

Overall, what you want to pay attention to is a combination of endurance (such as your walking program), flexibility (such as stretching or yoga to keep muscles supple and joints moving), and strength (some resistance exercises like weights so you can remain strong enough to take care of yourself).

Use of free weights is good, and better than static machines working a single muscle group. Today trainers recommend compound exercise movement to involve both the upper and lower body at the same time. This newer approach employs movements that feel natural as you use weights. Such combinations build muscle and burn calories faster than old exercise techniques. Compound exercises strengthen our core group of muscles and improve balance, both important for leverage movement in using arms and legs for day-to-day activities.

Balance is less commonly mentioned but disease, medication, even getting older can erode this vital function. When you were young you probably could stand on one foot with your eyes closed for 40 or more seconds. After age 60 many people can maintain such a pose for only a few seconds or not at all. Trainers today emphasize core exercises, use BOSU training programs and stability balls to improve balance and strength together. Balance can be improved. Within one month of starting the right program you will experience more strength, endurance, and flexibility. Measure what you can do now as baseline, like touching your toes or raising one arm over your head and trying to put your hand down behind your head to touch your backbone. Commit to having a professional trainer design a program and then make a month's effort. Retest yourself in 30 days. You'll see a difference!

What happens over time if you do not exercise is not good. A trainer friend of mine motivates his clients by telling them if they do not exercise they predictably will end life either in a wheelchair or using a walker. He cautions they will not have the strength to get in and out of a bath tub if they do not exercise.

Thousands of years ago the genetic ability to put on weight quickly was an advantage for prehistoric man. That may be why many of our ancestors survived and why you and I are here. But efficient weight gain now that food is plentiful ceases to be a competitive advantage. As you know, most people in America are either overweight or obese. The link between certain cancers such as colon and uterus and being overweight is clear. Disease prevention becomes another reason to pay attention to your weight. There are many formulas now to determine body composition such as the body mass index (BMI) for you to investigate. Here's a novel idea for you: instead of finding your height on a standard chart and looking across to see what an ideal weight would be, look instead at the weight chart first. Now, look back to see how tall you should be! Which will be easier for you to change, your weight or height?

In a way body fatness is a distraction. In the realm of cancer therapy we need to think more about how the proliferation of cancer cells is affected. Carcinogenesis, or how cancers establish their foothold, is the net effect of angiogenesis (new blood vessels supplying nutrients for the cancer), tumor cell proliferation, and apoptosis (what scientists say when they talk about cancer cells dying). It has been possible to show in colon cancer, and probably is true in others, exercise hastens tumor cell death.

A couple more pertinent facts: start with the observation that from prehistoric time until very recently our ancestors engaged in almost constant physical exertion to survive. This was true as recently as our grandparents or parents. It has come to light that in Victorian times, working class Englishmen commonly consumed more than 5000 calories a day without gaining weight because of the strenuous nature of daily life. Today even children do not get enough exercise and are getting fat.

John Medina in his book *Brain Rules* estimates primitive man traveled 12 miles a day searching for food or avoiding being eaten. Back then our ancestors were accustomed to constant change. If they stayed in one place more than a few minutes they might be detected and eaten. Dr. Medina deduces that even today that history survives in our genes. We learn better when moving because of that old experience. Our brains continue to be structurally altered by the very activity of exercise. In other words, movement produces a competitive advantage for us, affecting the success of everything we learn.

One attempt to quantify activity comes from measuring Physical Activity levels (PAL). If the energy to keep us alive at rest is given a numerical baseline value of 1.0, it can be estimated that a sedentary person watching television may have a PAL of only 1.15. For every 30 minutes of walking you can credit yourself with an additional 0.10 units. A PAL ratio of 1.7 or higher is judged sufficient for good health and has predictive value for some research. A low PAL combined with the average American diet is guaranteed to lead to weight gain.

Another useful measure to consider in your activity strategy is to remember the two main components of exercise are resistance and aerobics. These two are interrelated through Duration, Intensity, and Frequency factors, or DIF. As the sum effect of these three factors goes up, the risks to our health of cancer and cardiovascular disease go down. In reducing this to an equation, if we up the intensity of our exercise, either the duration or frequency factors can be reduced. In one study 17 minutes of brisk walking gave the same benefit as 30 minutes of leisurely stroll. If you choose an exercise that is less intense, work out longer or more often.

Just to mention a couple more rationales from a host of data on the benefit of exercise, we know that sustained exercise releases substances into the circulation that actually make us feel good. Less well recognized is the fact that chronic inflammation is linked to many diseases, including cancer. And by the way, fat tissue contains a high percentage of inflammatory cells, so that's another strike against obesity. A substance called cytokine IL-6 dramatically increases in the circulation after exercise. Cytokine IL-6 both reduces mediators that cause inflammation and increases anti-inflammatory mediators.

Aside from cancer, cardiovascular disease is the other major cause of premature death in this country. Dr. Bortz, mentioned in Chapter 8, is still running marathons and he is in his late 70s. He points out that all the angst about thread-sized coronary arteries becoming plugged, like we see on television commercial cartoons, would go away with an active program of running. "We could stop worrying about heart disease if we trained enough to have coronary arteries the size of garden hoses!" he once told me. You probably won't achieve that degree of success, but the benefits of running can grow out of a simple program of walking 30 minutes a day.

I need to be cautious because you the reader are unknown to me. I have no information about your fitness level. You need specific guidance from your physician, a professional trainer, or both. I do know of many occasions in my practice where I tried to assist someone chronically ill, maybe near death from cancer. I wrapped my fingers around an upper arm to give a lift and realized I held something twig-like, smaller than that person's wrist. No muscle remained, just skin and bone. That's the point where we become too weak to transfer from chair to bed or even go to the bathroom. Such a person is too frail to enjoy life anymore. It becomes a burden just to live. We suffer the final indignities of total dependence and the bed pan. From those experiences I am moved to write these cautionary observations. Don't let inactivity do this to you.

Almost every reader can take steps to avoid such a dismal outcome. Be proactive and start now. Work out what makes sense to you about combating cancer at the cellular level with good nutrition and other ideas in this book. Devise a way to mobilize your immune system and go on the offense. Visualize energy flowing through your circulation, killing cancer cells by the very act of exercising. And as this book has been telling you, utilize your intellect to learn, reduce stress, and join with others for mutual support.

So in exercise and all these things, as common sense would tell you, get started. Doing something to help your self is much better than nothing at all.

APPENDIX IV
BOOKS RECOMMENDED BY RENEWAL MEMBERS

Barnett, John, *How to Feel Good as You Age.* Acton, MA: VanderWyk & Burnham, 2000.

Courteney, Hazel, *500 of the Most Important Health Tips You'll Ever Need.* London: Cico Books, 2001.

Cousins, Norman, *Anatomy of an Illness.* New York: Norton and Company, Inc., 1979.

Cunningham, Alastair J., *Can the Mind Heal Cancer?* 2005.

Dossey, Larry, *Beyond Illness.* Boulder, CO: Shambhala, 1984.

Dossey, Larry, *Healing Words.* San Francisco: Harper, 1993.

Geffen, Jeremy R., *The Journey Through Cancer: An Oncologist's Seven-Level Program for Healing and Transforming the Whole Person.* New York: Random House, 2006.

Gonzales, Laurence, *Deep Survival.* New York: W.W. Norton, 2004.

Hay, Louise L., *You Can Heal Your Life.* Santa Monica, CA: Hay House, 1984.

Katz, Lawrence C., *Keep Your Brain Alive*. New York: Workman Publishing Co., 1999.

LeShan, L., *Cancer as a Turning Point*. New York: Dutton, 1989.

Mahmud, Khalid, *Keeping aBreast: Ways to Stop Breast Cancer*. Bloomington, IN: AuthorHouse, 2005.

Mathai, Kimberly and Ginny Scott, *The Cancer Lifeline Cookbook*. Seattle: Sasquatch Books, 2004.

Medina, John, *Brain Rules*. Seattle: Pear Press, 2008.

Moody, Raymond A., *The Light Beyond*. New York: Bantam Books, 1988.

Olson, James S., *Bathsheba's Breast: Women, Cancer, and History*. Baltimore: The Johns Hopkins University Press, 2002.

Pelletier, Kenneth R., *Mind as Healer Mind as Slayer*. New York: Dell, 1977.

Pollan, Michael, *The Omnivore's Dilemma*. Penguin Group USA, 2006.

Remen, Rachel Naomi, *Kitchen Table Wisdom: Stories That Heal*. New York: Riverhead Books, 1996.

Sattilaro, Anthony J., *Recalled by Life*. Boston: Houghton Mifflin, 1982.

Siegel, Bernie S., *Love, Medicine & Miracles*. New York: Harper & Row, 1986.

Siegel, Bernie S., *Peace, Love & Healing*. New York: Harper & Row, 1989.

Simonton, O. Carl, S. Matthews-Simonton and J. Creighton, *Getting Well Again*. New York: Bantam Books, 1978.

Simonton, O. Carl and R. Henson, *The Healing Journey*. New York: Authors Choice Press, 1992.

Szekely, Edmond B., *Guide to the Essene Way of Biogenic Living*. International Biogenic Society, 1977.

Tipping, Colin C., *Radical Forgiveness*. Marietta GA: Global 13 Publications, 1997.

West, Melissa Gayle, *Silver Linings: Finding Hope, Meaning and Renewal During Times of Transition*. Fair Winds Press, 2004.

Draw how I see my self and/or my problem or illness (cf pp. 32-3, 98). Create detail and use color if possible.

Diagram your issues and problems (cf pp. 168-9).

List people, actions to forgive (cf pp. 140-1, 258-9), affirmations (cf pp. 202-5), promises to my self (cf p. 164).

MY NOTES